VOLUME TO VALUE

PROVEN METHODS FOR ACHIEVING
HIGH QUALITY IN HEALTHCARE

VOLUME
TO VALUE

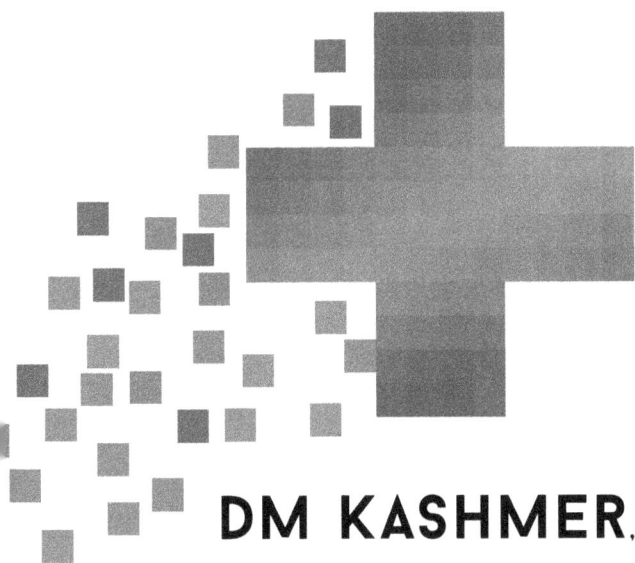

DM KASHMER, MD, MBA

VOLUME TO VALUE

Proven Methods for Achieving
High Quality in Healthcare

ISBN   978-1-61961-467-3 *Paperback*
        978-1-61961-468-0 *Ebook*

LIONCREST
PUBLISHING

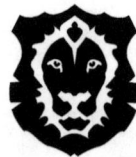

CONTENTS

FOREWORD

BY KIM HOLLON

The American health-care system is much more expensive than most industrialized countries, and improvements in our life expectancy have not kept pace with other countries. The causes for our lower value are complicated, in part because our system is complicated. Regardless of the systemic causes for our lack of significant progress, we will experience similar results over the next ten years if we do not change the way we lead our health-care system.

I believe that we face several fundamental structural barriers to positive change that are not within the scope of

control of the average provider. Our fee-for-service pay-
ment systems have not been aligned with creating value,
although this is changing within the country. Combine
the incentive for volume with a supply-side economic
system, with poor measures of quality and value, and with
a professional-knowledge-based management system,
and you get a system designed for our current outcomes.

Our professional-knowledge-based management system
places the individual clinician (physician, nurse, therapist, etc.) in charge of managing care delivery within this
very complex system. For example, in most hospitals,
the number of on-site managers falls by over 90 percent
sometime after 5:00 p.m. each day, with similar supervision on weekends. Combine this with very large spans
of control and physicians who have been trained to think
that they are individually responsible for crafting the
care delivery to the specific needs of their patients, and
you get a system with tremendous variability in process.

One leader cannot change all of the structural problems
in our system, but he or she can acknowledge them and
develop a system aimed at improving value within these
constraints. I believe the key to sustained improvements in
safety, quality, and value lies in engaging the front line in
careful examination and improvement of our culture and
processes. As a skilled surgeon, Dr. Kashmer daily experi-

ences the variability in our systems and has great insight into how we can improve from the inside. In this book, he merges the experience of a frontline staff member with advanced quality-improvement concepts such as the DMAIC pathway and the Box-Cox transformation to demonstrate how we can greatly improve healthcare using those powerful tools to help us along.

I know the practical wisdom shared in this book will provide examples of how we can improve the healthcare system.

—KIM HOLLON, FACHE
CEO, SIGNATURE HEALTHCARE

INTRODUCTION

Have you heard that the US Department of Health and Human Services (HHS) has set a goal of tying 50 percent of hospital reimbursement payments to quality/value by the end of 2018? If you *have* heard, are you *ready*?

If the costs of poor quality and patient outcomes weren't reasons enough to prepare for the coming changes in reimbursement, now we have this major new impetus to improve as we go from volume to value. Now, consider this question: Do you and your organization have a process to push out new (and more) quality endpoints as reimbursement changes?

This book shares *many* of the highly effective tools that are already well known in the field of quality improvement—tools that can be applied *directly* in healthcare. I've been doing just that in different teams for over fifteen years. Please consider this book as my opportunity to share with you some of the most effective ways to make that change from volume- to value-based care.

As a Lean Six Sigma master black belt, I've witnessed (and helped drive) healthcare's improved adoption of the Lean Six Sigma methodology. In this book, I explain some well-known tools, philosophies, and interventions that can help your system succeed as we all go through this important reimbursement transition. Remember, the Lean Six Sigma methodologies are tool sets. Even if you're not able to adopt this approach completely in your organization or practice, just reading about some of the standard quality-improvement tools these approaches string together will go a long way toward helping you with the issues we're all facing.

I look forward to where we are going in healthcare. I hope you find the tools in this work useful as a map that can guide you toward an improved focus on even higher quality—and more valuable—care.

PREFACE

Another blizzard had hit the city, and the hospital was snowed in—again. Staff coming off shift couldn't leave; incoming shifts couldn't get there. The hospital was crowded with people, but it was oddly quiet. All ambulatory surgery and medical appointments had been canceled, and very few new patients had been admitted during the storm.

The little café on the second floor was a favorite spot for staff members to grab a coffee and a snack. Because so many people were stuck at the hospital, it was unusually full that late afternoon, to the point where an administrator new to the hospital couldn't find an empty table. He asked the tired-looking guy in scrubs sitting at a corner table if they could share.

He apologized for not knowing the doctor's name. "I'm new here," he said. "I'm heading up the quality-improvement initiative, but I haven't had a chance to meet everyone yet." The doctor introduced himself as the head of the department of surgery. "I'm new here, too. I'm really glad to meet you. Quality improvement is my passion. I'm actually a Lean Six Sigma master black belt."

"Really? You're a master black belt? So that means you've helped whole organizations deploy Lean Six Sigma and that you mentor project leaders, right? I studied Lean Six Sigma when I was getting my MBA, but I couldn't figure out how to apply it to healthcare. Eliminating defects on a production line just doesn't seem as if it would translate well into a people-centered hospital setting."

"You'll be amazed at how well it works," replied the surgeon. "Let me tell you about this great project we did at my last job..."

Two hours later, the snow was still falling. The new administrator and the surgeon were now allies in the cause of health-care quality improvement using statistical process control. They agreed to meet weekly in the café to compare notes and continue their discussion.

CHAPTER 1

WHY BOTHER WITH ADVANCED QUALITY TOOLS?

The blizzard had passed, and life at the big hospital had returned to its normal bustle. The surgeon and the hospital administrator met for a quiet coffee to catch up. The administrator was starting to understand the basic concepts of the Lean Six Sigma approach, but he was still skeptical. "Why," he asked the surgeon, "should we bother with advanced quality tools? Surely we're smart enough to see right away what the problems are, fix them, and just assume that a fix means saving money. It's really hard to get the accounting guys to tell me how much we're saving—I'm not so sure they really know anyway. Why go through all the work of data collection, statistical analysis, and all that other math stuff?"

The surgeon replied, "I see your point about making quality improvement more complicated than it has to be, but all you have to do is look at the typical project to see that we need more than our gut feelings to assess what the problem really is. I can tell you right now that the average quality improvement project in healthcare saves about $250,000. But there's more to it than that. We need to know not only how much a project saves in actual costs but also what it saves in terms of the cost of poor quality. Let me tell you about the case of the misfiring stapler and what it turned out to really cost..."

+ + +

At the large medical center where I previously worked, we have a great surgeon who is particularly skilled in laparoscopic techniques. A big part of Dr. Smith's success, particularly with elective procedures, is that he always does things exactly the same way, deviating only when he absolutely has to. He has surgery down to a very efficient science—and he has great outcomes. But one day he arrived in the operating room to find that the type of surgical stapler he had used very successfully for more than a decade had been replaced by a new model from a different manufacturer. The thinking from the hospital administration was that the new stapler was less expensive and would work just as well. It was indeed cheaper, and it really did work as well, but it wasn't as simple for Dr. Smith to use, in part because it was new to the team. His scrub tech loaded it incorrectly, but Dr. Smith couldn't tell that from looking at it. When he fired, the staple load ejected out of the end. The anastomosis he was going for wasn't created correctly, and he had to dig around in the patient to find the ejected staple load. He couldn't salvage the situation—the laparoscopy had to turn into a laparotomy. The procedure took significantly longer; the patient remained hospitalized for an extra day. Fortunately, no complications developed.

Lots of questions emerge from Dr. Smith's experience. At the micro level, should operating rooms (ORs) be able to mandate the equipment surgeons use? Should ORs change equipment without consulting the surgeons? Should the surgeons be able to decide everything, and if not, how much should they be able to decide?

More importantly, questions arise at the macro level. What are the costs associated with decisions such as these? How do we capture what this event costs? What is the cost of poor quality?

The answers to these questions matter. In the immediate sense, they help guide us when it comes to decisions about switching equipment or changing procedures. In the broader sense, when we do a quality-improvement project in a hospital, how much do we think we're actually saving? Cheaper staplers aren't a savings if outcomes are worse down the line. Over time, it turns out that the highest quality outcomes are actually the cheapest. The highest quality systems are in fact cheaper and better. They minimize the severe costs associated with poor quality.

How do we figure out what quality costs? And when we say cost, to whom is that cost directed? To the patient? To the hospital? To the third-party payer? If something happens in the OR, and you have to convert the surgery to a laparotomy instead of using the camera, the third-party payer will still reimburse you for the procedure. If they're still going to pay you for the procedure, then how do you calculate what the cost of that quality issue was?

USING LEAN SIX SIGMA

Lean Six Sigma answers hard questions in healthcare by applying data to them. Lean Six Sigma is a data-driven method used by organizations of all kinds to improve their performance and reduce errors and defects. The system basically "strings together" a number of well-known quality-improvement tools. It's not as if the term Lean Six

Sigma applies only to manufacturing processes, where it refers to producing a very low number of defective products on a production line, or having very close to no variation from one item to the next so that every widget is exactly the same. The Lean approach and Six Sigma statistical-thinking approach may have begun at manufacturing companies such as Motorola, Westinghouse, and Toyota, but they're easily applicable to processes and systems involving people who need to use their judgment and experience to make decisions. Because the system involves logical thinking, the use of well-validated tools, and a systematic approach to problem-solving, Lean Six Sigma (which uses both Lean and Six Sigma tools) takes a lot of the guesswork and individual bias out of quality-improvement projects in healthcare. That may sound a bit impersonal, but in fact the system encourages initiative, imagination, and unorthodox solutions. Lean Six Sigma projects are designed to save time and money, eliminate waste, reduce errors, improve efficiency, and keep patients safe. These proven tools can help us progress from a health-care system based on the *volume* of care provided to one focused on the *value* of care delivered.

THE COPQ TOOL

High-quality healthcare is cheaper in the long run. As Dr. Smith's patient shows, the cost of an extra day in the hospital obviates all the savings from using a different stapler on that case. Similarly, rushing a patient out of the hospital before they're really ready to go home can lead to readmission and a subsequent Medicare penalty.

In Lean Six Sigma, we use a tool called the Cost of Poor Quality (COPQ) to quantify how much money can be recovered or saved by a health-care quality project. This is a great tool for making the business case for the project. Of course, the COPQ is really a measure of waste owing to poor quality. But it helps that it's a measure that turns waste into a dollar amount.

The costs of poor quality can be visualized by imagining four different buckets.

1. **Internal failures.** These are failures in the process that have a cost but don't directly affect the end user. Is the end user the patient or the third-party payer? This is a challenging question that can make it difficult to determine the COPQ for internal failures.

2. **External failures.** These are failures in the process that do directly affect the patient and prolong the hospital stay.

3. **Surveillance.** When the quality of systems is poor, they end up requiring costly increased surveillance from state regulatory bodies, accrediting agencies, and so on. Often,

the hospital has to pay an accrediting body to come survey the hospital. Poor quality can lead to, for example, extra surveys—which are costly.

4. **Prevention.** Spending money on preventing problems is the one quality element that has a clear positive return on investment. Prevention has a multiplier effect because it prevents internal, external, and surveillance-related issues.

GETTING NUMBERS TO CRUNCH

The finance department in the hospital has to be willing to be transparent with their data. They have to be willing to look openly at the profit-and-loss statement with you and decide what costs are incurred under each bucket. Or, in other words, what costs are incurred by poor quality? And, don't forget, if you're being reimbursed right now for additional care, you have to work even harder to surpass what income you are receiving because of your poor quality. For example, if you're still paid for an intensive-care-unit (ICU) stay that occurred because you gave a patient the wrong medication, you need to make sure everyone knows those additional revenues will disappear after you eliminate the quality issue you're working on!

Two other financial factors need to be considered in the cost of poor quality. First, the increased risk of potential liability arising from poor quality is a real possibility. Second, defects in care lead to lower reimbursement recovery from Medicaid, Medicare, and other third-party payers. The cost of this can be very high. Let's say that an external failure means a catheter gets left too long in a patient and causes a urinary-tract infection (UTI) on the eighth day of a hospitalization. It's possible that the defect means no reimbursement to the hospital at all for fees related to that patient's care.

THE TRUE COST OF POOR QUALITY

That's why the COPQ is such a useful construct to figure out. What does poor quality cost? Usually, it's a surprisingly high amount.

The COPQ is challenging for the finance department, because students aren't taught about it in accounting or MBA courses. There's no line item for the cost of poor quality. The only way to figure it out is to work with the finance people to draw it out from the core accounting, particularly the profit-and-loss statements. It's tough to draw the line between indirect and direct poor quality costs—they're hard to quantify. Where do you draw the line between hard savings and softer savings? The conservative way to do it is to say, "We expect that if we fix these quality issues, we're going to save X dollars."

SHORTENING THE STAY

Shortening the length of a hospital stay is generally seen as desirable. Costs are lower, the risk of hospital-related infection is reduced, and patients recover better at home. But rushing a patient out of the hospital or discharging someone prematurely can lead to readmission, which can carry a very high cost in lost reimbursement and patient risk.

Quality programs that include shorter hospital stays have to incorporate metrics that show the downside. If you shorten the typical length of stay, but your readmission rate goes through the roof, is that really effective? You have to consider readmissions as you decide on your quality endpoints.

Statistical process-control tools can be used to analyze this. In the data-collection plan, you build in a realistic sample size so you can tell when you're doing better or worse. You have to determine how big a sample you need to show some meaningful change. The endpoints should measure what really matters.

OPERATIONAL DEFINITIONS

In the case of length of stay, both length of stay and readmission rate have an operational definition. An operational definition is the definition you and the team either create or accept for the purposes of your project. Let me tell you, the operational definition for an endpoint affects *a lot*.

Among other things, creating an operational definition means defining when the clock starts. That might seem simple, the sort of thing everybody just knows, yet I've learned from experience that the definition of length of stay, for example, can be all over the map. Does it mean from the time the order goes in to admit the patient until the discharge order goes in? That definition seems to make perfect sense, but not everybody does it that way. Consider that even once the patient is officially discharged, he or she may still physically be in the hospital. The patient might not have a ride home, for example, so he or she is still physically in a bed. The bed can't be cleaned, and the room can't be made ready for another patient. So which operational definition will you choose? One that focuses on orders going into a computer or one that focuses on when a patient actually leaves? You can see how important an operational definition is during a project.

What's valuable about statistical process-control tools, particularly those of Lean Six Sigma, is that they force you as a group to come up with clear operational definitions for what the heck you're talking about, such as when the clock starts and when it stops. When someone comes to the emergency room (ER), when has she actually arrived? When she walks through the door, or when she first checks in with the triage nurse? Or when she first gets led back to a treatment bay? What if an ambulance brings her? What if she is shot and then dropped off in front of your ER? What definition is most meaningful needs to be decided before a quality-improvement project begins. Otherwise, changes are made and no difference is seen in the data, because the change isn't being measured by that data.

QUALITY SAVINGS

The median recovery on a quality-improvement project is an astoundingly high $250,000. This is one way to measure the cost of poor quality. One successful project to reduce urinary-tract infections could bring in a quarter of a million dollars in direct savings. This should inspire a willingness to spend money on quality, but typically it doesn't. Most people in healthcare simply aren't aware of this particular statistic. The focus tends to be much more on concerns about money being withheld if certain endpoints aren't improved. In meeting after meeting, we hear about how much money we're going to "lose." When I worked at one hospital, I actually did the math. I found that for an organization of our size, the amount of "lost" money worked out to be about $180,000 for the year. If the median recovery of a quality-improvement project is much more than that, why not just do the project?

Government in the form of Medicaid and Medicare is very visible to people in healthcare. It's easy for them to see if the hospital is "losing" money from withheld reimbursements. It's a lot harder to see that the hospital is losing that amount (and more) every day in small amounts from multiple pockets, because perhaps the hospital doesn't know, or even acknowledge the existence of, the cost of poor quality.

Once you use the COPQ tool, however, you can easily see that you have a plethora of possible quality-improvement projects that you could do. They range from the very difficult to the very easy. Any one of those projects could recover just as much or even a lot more than might be withheld. It's amazing what can be recovered if the focus is on true quality-improvement projects and not just on strengthening reimbursement from the government.

TRUE QUALITY IMPROVEMENT

Distinguishing between worthwhile projects that will provide true quality improvement and those that won't is easier if you apply DMAIC, a core approach of Lean Six Sigma. DMAIC stands for define, measure, analyze, improve, and control. (I'll go into this in more detail in chapter 4.) For now, let's look at the *define* phase. It's a systematic way to solve a problem or improve a process. It's helpful to think of DMAIC as a cycle—it's not necessarily a linear process.

That's where we make the project charter and discuss who needs to be involved with the project, who the stakeholders are, what the problem is, and what the cost of poor quality is for the project. We figure all that out, and we put it up front to make it visible.

The beauty of the DMAIC process is that, because it puts data first, some of what emerges is often counterintuitive. In a project to reduce urinary-tract infections in hospitalized patients, for example, the *define* stage may reveal that a lot of patients are actually coming into the hospital with existing UTIs. Many patients arrive at the hospital from nursing homes and have indwelling catheters. When the define stage reveals how many patients come in with infections, it can change the focus of your quality-improvement project. The original thought might have been to train nurses better in inserting catheters. Instead, the better project might be to identify patients who already have a UTI when they arrive at the hospital. The Lean Six Sigma process keeps you from defining your intervention ahead of your data.

We have a tendency in healthcare to decide that we know what the problem is because we live it every day. But we're not objective, and we don't see the whole picture, only our little part of it. Lean Six Sigma makes you question every assumption by putting data on it. It takes nothing for granted. Most healthcare defects are complex and multifactorial. Lean Six Sigma helps embody the complexity. The holes in the Swiss cheese don't line up to make a defect.

For a group that's used DMAIC before, the median time for getting a quality-improvement project underway and seeing results is thirty to sixty days. The projects don't drag on for a year and fall apart with incomplete results. Early on, however, DMAIC projects can take *much* longer.

SAVINGS FROM COPQ

In the context of a massive hospital budget that runs to many millions of dollars, saving $250,000 from a single project may not sound like much. But it's real money that could be the salaries for multiple advanced practitioners or additional nurses, or for renovating the waiting area in the ER, or for some other project that's on a back burner for lack of funding. And if you were to implement three different quality-improvement projects in the course of a year, and each one saved you $250,000, now we're talking serious money.

The cost of implementing each quality-improvement project is hard to guess ahead of time. You may not get all the interventions you want, because some may just be too expensive. I always try to see how much bang I can get for my buck by playing the hand that I'm dealt. One way to evaluate interventions is by intensity. How hard are they, how expensive are they, and how practically applicable are they? In the case of reducing UTIs, an effective intervention is to automatically do a urinalysis on every patient who arrives from a nursing home with a catheter. This turns out to be an excellent intervention: the cost is very, very low; getting the sample is very simple and very quick. The payoff in terms of getting the patient diagnosed and treatment started quickly is high. These sorts of small, powerful interventions are the best because they work so well. Everybody can see how effective they are; they get on board and make sure they're done every time.

The tools I'll talk about in this book embrace complexity and give good answers. In the case of Dr. Smith's (really the patient's) stapler problem, they ask the right questions: What were the real ramifications of the stapler misfire? What were the true costs? What kind of intervention should we consider to avoid this ever happening again? How much is that intervention worth? What would the world look like if we didn't intervene? The COPQ can tell us, at a system level at least, how much waste we have in a given system and what we may be able to reclaim when we make improvements.

Typically, people don't think about the true costs associated with true quality. Even if they do start to think about them, they think only in the near term of how much money was saved in a year by switching to a different stapler. A more robust view is that these are the actual costs associated with a quality issue. Rather than apply the costs to one event, apply it to the whole system, and get a sense of what the overall costs and savings from a quality-improvement project will be. When we apply the costs of poor quality over entire systems and project those costs over hundreds of patients, we get a much better sense of how much to invest in fixing a quality issue.

PENNY-WISE

When a system doesn't recognize the true costs of doing things poorly, it can choose interventions that save pennies by cutting or restricting things and completely miss interventions that could save lots of dollars. It's all too easy not to recognize the cost to the whole system as a problem.

I once had to figure out a good intervention to a problem with medication dispensing in a hospital. Administering the wrong dose of a drug, or prescribing a drug that a patient was known to be allergic to, was happening far too often. Problems like these carry serious risks to the patient and to the system. If a patient is made worse from a wrong dose or allergic reaction, the length of stay could be increased by days. And if the patient dies, the consequences to the system could be severe. It's easy to see how high the cost of poor quality is when it comes to medication errors.

Why was this happening? In fact, once upon a time the pharmacy department was overstaffed and costing more than it should. But in the effort to reduce the staff, the administrative team overshot and laid off too many people, including the person in charge of overseeing quality in the pharmacy. Understaffing can be as expensive as overstaffing if the staff is reduced so low that quality suffers. The pharmacy department budget looked better, but the system was actually incurring way more expense from the cost of poor quality. Similar things happen a lot because, after all, a department profit-and-loss statement has no column that shows how much bad quality is costing the system.

We incurred huge unforeseen costs by cutting a linchpin position. This unfortunate, costly, dangerous situation could have been avoided by more careful evaluation before the position was cut, but, again, the COPQ is not written in bright red ink on a profit-and-loss statement. It's not easy to see how much poor quality costs. In this case, the problem was easy to solve: bring back the laid-off quality manager. Of course, there were other options, but in that particular case that's the one the team decided to implement once they realized how the now-visible COPQ problem was *much* more costly than the position had been. Even better than the solution to have an employee who checks to make sure there's no quality issue would be for the team to design a system that didn't make as many defects and so didn't need as much surveillance.

MEASURABLE CHANGE

Too often, a team puts a lot of time and effort into a quality-improvement project that seems to make a difference, only to be told by the C-suite that they're not seeing any of the savings that the COPQ tool promised. When you are making a cost estimate for a quality-improvement project, working with your financial group—the chief financial officer (CFO) or delegate—is crucial for success. You have to come up with a realistic estimate of the tangible savings that you can reasonably expect from the project. The financial group has to agree. In my experience, it's far better to be collaborative with your finance team than it is to overpromise and underdeliver. This can be a problem, because it's hard to be rigorous if the financial people don't want to share the data. Some don't want to share just on principle, but often they can't share, because they're not really sure what the data are or that you'll understand it even if they give it to you. Will you understand the context the data fit into? Will you (or even should you) understand their overall financial plan for the health system? That's why collaboratively looking at the financial data is so key. It puts everyone on the same page. Do it early and often as you make a COPQ estimate.

Another classic reason quality projects fail is "scope creep." In some surveys of project failures, scope creep is the single most common reason for failure. The project just keeps getting bigger and bigger, to the point where it's almost certain to fail.

An additional important cause of project failure is poor or no root causation. Perhaps the group never really had an honest conversation about what the root issues are. Those issues may have been politically sensitive, so they got swept under the rug. If you need to have a crucial conversation and you don't have it for whatever reason, that's a problem. You never find the true root cause for the issue you're studying. You don't measure what you need to. Failure ensues.

Here's another reason for failure: poor or no champion

involvement. Every project needs a champion, someone who is committed to the culture change the project will make happen. A champion keeps the project moving forward by working out problems and keeping the team enthusiastic and committed. The ideal champion is usually a stakeholder from the C-suite. This person can get you and the team the resources you need. That could be as simple as arranging for a conference room when you've been told none is available to something as complex as getting you the resources to do a computer system sweep.

Projects can also fail if the stakeholders, or at least some of them, aren't in the room. These are the people who will have to participate in the project. If they're excluded or included only in a token way, the project won't get support from the participants. In my experience, any of the above issues doom a project to failure before the first DMAIC step is ever taken.

I once worked for an organization that, for a lot of complex political reasons, could never even mention that the emergency department could do a better job. When a quality-improvement project was set up, and a champion from the C-suite was named, the champion didn't even attend meetings, much less do anything to push the project forward. The project was dead in the water from the time it was first proposed.

Lean Six Sigma questions everything, which means it often runs up against sacred cows. Often, it can tip the cow over, but not always. Quality improvement, in some organizations, may even be framed as a fight, but it's not. In other organizations, it's a culture change that is moving the system to an attitude of everyone wanting to constantly improve. If that attitude isn't there, or if the attitude is to leave things alone as long as they're working reasonably well, it's very hard to make headway with Lean Six Sigma—or any process-improvement system. The precondition for success is that the organization may already feel it's world-class, but also feel that it can always do better. If that attitude isn't there, then it's difficult to even start down the path of moving from a volume mentality to a value mentality.

Corporate culture matters and can be deeply entrenched. Over the years, I've worked with groups whose attitudes ranged from "We're perfect, so don't bother us," to "Oh my god, everything's wrong, hair on fire, let's fix everything," to "Well, we think we're really, really good, but maybe there's just a little room to improve." Even that last one had great success with quality-improvement projects.

If you think everything is close to perfect in your organization, and someone shows you an objective measurement that says it isn't, you might still ignore it. The power of the human mind to see only what it wants to see is amazing. There are a lot of ways to frame the denial. You can just flat-out deny it; you can say there's nothing wrong; you can say the data are false; you can say the data have been manipulated; you can personally attack the person who brings you the data; you can say a personal or political agenda is driving the data. That last accusation should, incidentally, be true. If your goal is to improve the center and, most importantly, your care for patients, then yes, you do have an agenda, and, yes, that is driving the data.

People can have a very hard time reacting well to data about performance when those data are unpalatable. I think it's because the information is so out of their frame sometimes that they'll do everything they can to reframe it, including saying that it's not true, that's not how it is, and you, as the person presenting the information, are a terrible person. To a degree, you have to expect being called everything from a bully to a jerk. As the change agent, you're in a tough spot. People often just hate change, and they may even take it out on you. No matter how collegial and transparent you are, no matter how sincerely you say, "Look, it's about our improving together with data," people are afraid they're going to lose face within the organization or even lose their jobs. Remember, things are the way they are in organizations for *reasons*. The organization is aligned around the way things are *before* any changes are made.

So, building a philosophy that "we use data in teams to improve as a group" is probably *the* key factor. Adopting that mind-set means that data will be used to decide on changes and improvements. That the data will be collected and interpreted by a *team* means that there is no (or at least little) us-versus-them mentality that holds so many organizations back.

BLACK BELTS AND PROJECT CHARTERS

For a quality-improvement project to succeed, it needs to start with a good interdisciplinary team. That team's first task is to make up a project charter. This document lays out the nature of the project and defines exactly what you're working to accomplish. It defines the stakeholders, the scope of the project, and the cost of poor quality.

A quality-improvement project is a team sport that relies on stakeholders to play their parts. The project charter should be clear from the start about the involved parties and their roles. In the absence of a strong team, there can be no quality improvement.

The scope of the project is key to success. The scope should be very clear about the starting and stopping points for the project and what the focus should be. Again, one of the most common causes of project failure is scope creep: the project expands and becomes too large, with too many elements.

The COPQ is important here, because it gives the bottom-line expected return on the quality-improvement project.

In Lean Six Sigma, someone on the team is designated as the tour guide for the project, better known as the black belt. This is the person who will get the team together and guide them through the steps of the quality project. Usually, that person is an outside consultant or someone educated in-house who is trained in Lean Six Sigma techniques and who is able to do the statistical number crunching that's at the heart of the project.

It's up to the black belt to put the team together. In some organizations, if the black belt says you're on the team, then you're on the team—it's not a request. Other organizations rely on volunteers for teams. If you've already had some early successes, it's easier to talk people into joining. If there's no previous example, people are often a little suspicious. They wonder if the project will be worth their time and effort, or even if it will turn into some sort of witch hunt. The first meeting usually involves a slideshow to explain what the goals are, what the steps will be, and what participating will mean for the individuals. A good slideshow goes a long way to reassure everyone on the value of volunteering.

Unfortunately, the team members are almost always expected to do the project in addition to what they're already doing. Usually, they're not offered any protected time. If your philosophy as a health-care provider is that quality is just one more thing that you're stuck with doing, you won't get much out of participating. But if you think quality is the most important thing in medicine, then investing your time in the project will be worthwhile in itself. When you collect data, or even pull patient charts after the fact to look at what went wrong, that's not a waste of time. That could keep you from repeating the same mistake. These quality-improvement meetings prevent defects. The quality improvements you help implement will save you time down the line. And they'll help you give your patients better care. In the end, that's why you're in medicine.

Despite all the hard work people put in on these projects, they often don't even get much credit for them. Maybe at the end of the project there's an expression of thanks through a pizza party, but usually they don't even get that level of recognition from management. I make a real effort to recognize the people on the team. I send out regular updates that highlight individual contributions. I thank everybody all the time. I make sure credit is given where it's due. When I'm asked about team participants for things such as annual reviews, I report very favorably on what they've done.

Another approach that really helps bring people aboard is twofers: I try to align the quality-improvement project with other endpoints that are relevant to them. In the data-collection plans (I'll talk more about that in chapter 6), we try to select some endpoints that team members have on their radar, too. Twofers align the group's success with individual successes. This incentivizes the individuals to really participate, because what the group is doing is in part something they were going to have to do anyway by themselves. They actually can get it done with the group.

Groups seem to work best when they have between five and ten people, depending on the scope of the project and the number of stakeholders. If the group is any larger than ten, you get into the bystander effect, where some people don't contribute. Usually you need to get just one stakeholder from each group who has the ability and interest to make things stick. If you're doing a project that will impact respiratory therapy, surgery, and radiology, you need to get one person from each group, preferably someone who's empowered to make decisions. You don't want to reconvene the group over and over, and you don't want to have them bring decisions to their managers to get permission to make the change. You want people in the room who can make the changes the group decides upon.

The black belt's job is to get the group where it needs to go. It's not really to decide anything; it's just to get the group to use the tools of Lean Six Sigma and find the solutions in response to meaningful data. The black belts don't decide ahead of time what the changes are going to be. Instead, they help the group decide what tools to use and then show them how to use the tools effectively. After changes are made, a black belt helps demonstrate whether there's been a significant improvement and helps design the way in which the process will be monitored in an ongoing fashion to make sure it doesn't go off the rails. In the end, keeping everybody marching forward is the main job for the black belt.

WHERE DO I START?

The administrator and the surgeon met again for coffee in the little second-floor café. By now, the administrator was starting to feel at home in the hospital. He was getting the hang of the computer system, and he could find his way to most places without getting lost.

When the surgeon asked him what he'd been up to the past week, the administrator replied, "I've been meeting with department heads to talk to them about their ideas for quality-improvement projects. They sure have a lot of them."

The surgeon replied, "I know. I can see a lot of possibilities just in the department of surgery. My residents have some pretty good ideas."

"So does everyone," said the administrator. "Some are so good and simple that I don't know why they haven't been done already. A couple are so different that I can't decide if they're totally brilliant or totally crazy. But mostly, I'm hearing a lot of ideas that sound like they might work, but I can't really tell if they'll work well enough to make them worthwhile."

"This whole move from volume to value is new to everyone, so I suggest looking for a project that will give good results quickly," the surgeon replied. "In my experience, that's a good way to kick things off and build support for the whole quality initiative."

The administrator agreed. "Good point about picking some low-hanging fruit to get things started. I can see several possibilities, but is there a way to decide which projects are most likely to succeed?"

"There is," said the surgeon. "Lean Six Sigma has a great tool called Failure Mode and Effects Analysis that's really helpful for prioritizing quality-improvement projects. The Failure part makes it sound negative, but it actually helps you decide which projects have the most potential value. Sometimes the answer isn't what you think it should be."

✛   ✛   ✛

In a teaching hospital, the administration asks surgery residents to do quality projects all the time. Anyone who comes into the organization, such as a head of a department, can see areas for quality-improvement projects. In fact, that's often why the person was brought in to begin with. In these situations, the question is, where do we start? Which project should we do first? Which project is going to have the greatest impact on the medical staff? Which will help patients the most?

Deciding what to do first actually has several dimensions. One is just the severity of the problem—that's very intuitive. Another is how common the problem is, which is usually intuitive as well. Another is deciding which project has the most value—and that's not always intuitive at all. In fact, the project with the most value may be hidden from view, even though it's the main reason a system needs repairs. Think of a key pipe in your house. It's behind a wall, so you can't see it or check on its condition easily. As long as it's working, you don't notice it. But if it breaks, you might not find out until a lot of damage is done.

THE FMEA TOOL

A great tool for highlighting problems you might not ordinarily think of is Failure Mode and Effects Analysis, or FMEA. FMEA is a Lean Six Sigma tool designed to prioritize potential projects on the basis of how they might fail. The tool ranks potential failure modes according to their severity, on a score of one to ten. If the outcome that a situation (or the project to repair it) could give is bad or worse, it receives a high severity score.

FMEA also ranks failure modes according to their probability of occurrence. If something is more likely to go wrong, or is already going wrong a lot, a project to fix it gets a higher score.

In the health-care setting, some defects are almost impossible to detect before they reach the patient. I like to paraphrase that old puzzle from philosophy class and ask, "If a defect happens in the forest...?" Perhaps some will say, "Well, the defect didn't really harm the patient, and it was almost impossible to detect in advance. Let's just not worry about this one." Here is the Lean Six Sigma way of looking at this: If it's difficult to detect the defect, then the defect matters even more. If there's no known way to detect the defect before it gets to the patient, that means it's even more important to prioritize that failure mode when using the FMEA tool. A defect you can't see and have a great deal of difficulty preventing is a ten on the FMEA parameter scale.

FMEA may be used to help pick the project that most needs

to be done, which is not necessarily the one that's most likely to succeed. Now, when you first start doing quality projects with the tools in this book, you may want to go for the low-hanging fruit, the obvious projects that have a very good chance of succeeding. You want to have early successes and highlight them. That's actually a good idea for establishing the value of quality-improvement projects, but once you get past the first couple easy projects, you really need what FMEA does. The FMEA tool tells you, of the set of ten quality projects that could make you busy, which one you should start with first in terms of bang for the buck. That project may not, of course, be the easiest one to get done. FMEA points you to the project that's the biggest deal in terms of straight-up addressing your quality issues.

Some projects, of course, are so obvious and have such straightforward, easy fixes that they fall into the "just do it" category. They don't take a committee. FMEA is much less relevant to those. An example might be when, in the course of another project, you realize along the way that a policy you're responsible for is just so old that it's out of date and needs to be revised to get it into compliance. Just do it. Or there might be a quality issue in the OR that's an easy fix just by changing the number of sutures on hand. In my experience, these types of easy fixes come up on a regular basis. You need to be alert for them and willing to act quickly.

TAKE YOUR PICK

A common quality-improvement scenario is when a colleague or manager comes to you and says, "Here are five things that need fixing; take your pick." That's exactly what FMEA is designed to do. FMEA isn't a one-person process—it's collaborative. So when you get those five suggestions, start by collaborating. Ask questions that will let you figure out what the key factors in each project are.

Question one is, how big a problem do you think this is? What *big* almost always refers to is the financial impact, but other issues, such as employee satisfaction or patient safety, could come into play. Asking this question will educate you about what the organization considers important. Ask the administrator to rank each problem on a scale of one to ten. (FMEA is made simpler by using standard templates with prefabricated scales that you can easily download, such as this one from the American Society for Quality: http://bit.ly/1glYwwy.) The discussion is a valuable part of the process, because you're building consensus and prioritizing. In some organizations, everything is a ten. All the problems are severe and urgent. You may have to get past some unrealistic thinking to prioritize the projects.

Next, figure out the probability of the problem. How common is it? What's the probability that it will happen?

If it's something that happens every day and you can't get away from it, that's a ten. If it's less frequent, then it's lower on the index. The problem, of course, is that you often don't have any way of knowing the numeric probability of a problem. You can make up for the lack of data by having conversations with the administration and getting the opinions of people familiar with the problem. You get a better sense of how common things are, and you also involve the people you report to.

The severity of the problem also needs to be evaluated. What's the worst possible outcome? (Perhaps it's catastrophic failure leading to patient death or permanent loss of function.) What's the least harmful outcome? (Maybe it's a near miss that the patient doesn't even realize happened.) Most problems will be somewhere in between. Work with the most likely outcome, not the worst-case scenario. Ranking the severity of outcomes on a scale of one to five is a good approach. In the absence of statistical data, talk with people and use your best judgment.

Detection, also called surveillance, is often the hardest part of FMEA. What's the probability of detecting a problem or failure? Some will be caught right away—maybe the failure triggers an alarm or a warning screen. Others will take a little or a lot longer to be noticed, and some may never be noticed at all. Once again, the likelihood of detection gets ranked from one to five. How high the detection ranking is for a problem should be counter-intuitive. The problem that will be seen almost at once doesn't rank very high. It's the subtle problem, the one that's tough to find, that should get prioritized. I find that's very valuable for me as a reminder. It makes me stop and think, "Wait a minute. I'll never be able to figure out this problem, so that's more important."

Finally, there's the dormancy period or latency of the problem. How long will this problem be a sleeper? Will someone find it during the same shift, or will it not be noticed for month? Again, this is one of these issues where you may not really have any information. Ask people about their experiences to try to get an idea.

Once you've figured out all the parameters, plugging the numbers into an FMEA template makes it fairly easy to decide which project to do. Any failure that's likely to result in catastrophic or major harm to a patient is a good place to start. So is any failure that happens quite often. If the failure has the potential for harming a patient and occurs often, fixing it is a top-priority project.

Sometimes the answer to which project comes first isn't as obvious. That's when it's helpful to do the math in the template. To get the risk score, multiply probability times severity times "surveillability." The composite risk score becomes self-explanatory. Compare the scores for the various possible projects, and carve off the one with the highest score. That's the one to attack first.

Or is it? Some organizations have sacred cows or political minefields—sometimes you just can't go where the risk score leads you, even if it's very high. Once those projects have been eliminated, look at what's left, and ask your group, "What can we achieve? This problem may be the biggest one to solve, but can we get there? What support will we need? Can we get it?"

Using the FMEA tool is almost like having a negotiation. It's invaluable for getting a sense of what the organization finds important.

FMEA SURPRISES

Sometimes a high risk score is a surprise. FMEA can end up giving you a counterintuitive answer. It sometimes says what you thought isn't the most important project actually is the most important project. What makes FMEA so valuable is that it's usually right. At one hospital where I worked, we had a very common problem we ran into every day. When patients came out of the OR, they were moved to the postanesthesia care unit (PACU). We were having a problem with the releasing orders for these patients getting backed up and being incomplete. We thought these frequent glitches in the paperwork flow were a big deal that could affect patient safety. At the same time, we were having issues of perioperative evaluation for blood typing and crossmatching that were much more severe but also much less common. The PACU issue was so in front of us all the time that it kept us from dealing with the perioperative issue. Also, the perioperative issue was hard to detect—we couldn't surveil for it, until it happened and we got into a bad situation because we hadn't done proper blood matching for the patient. We had a problem where we transfused blood that was not appropriate for the patient.

When that event happened, it actually took us in a totally different direction and made us focus on preoperative labs and how we could know when they hadn't come back, and especially how we could know whether the type and cross had been done. We were able to solve a problem we didn't even know we had. Fixing it wasn't even a big project. All we had to do was fix what the FMEA told us to fix.

If we didn't have a tool like FMEA, problems would be a lot harder to detect and solve. In medicine, we're very easily distracted by what's going on at the moment. It's very hard for an overworked administrator and the busy Chief of Surgery to get together. The administrator is rightfully focused on the complaints he or she keeps getting every day. If the administration is getting ten complaints a day about the same issue, the issue is important because it's common. Let's say the complaint is that too many beds are left in the hallway. That seems like a big deal because they clog up the corridors and people are literally running into them. At the same time, some patients aren't getting blood when they need it in a timely fashion. This is a more severe but less common problem. FMEA helps us prioritize and agree.

Without FMEA, a quality project to fix the bed problem may take priority over the blood problem. In fact, no one might even realize that there is a blood problem. With FMEA, the blood problem is uncovered because it has a high risk score. The FMEA tool may show the blood issue is the bigger deal and needs more attention. In fact, the bed problem probably doesn't need a quality project to be fixed. It's inconvenient, but patients are unlikely to be harmed by it—this falls into the "just do it" category of fixes. It might be as simple as reshuffling the shift assignments of the patient-transport staff.

FINDING FAILURE

Why is it so hard to see the signs that something is going wrong in a system? Why is it so hard to figure out if you have a problem? FMEA was first developed to detect technical failures and manufacturing defects in things like shipbuilding and assembly lines, where the human element isn't really that important. When it's applied to services such as healthcare, a lot of other issues get in the way and make it more difficult to detect things. Often it's internal politics or interest groups that can't even be discussed.

Systems, especially (I've found) emergency surgery and trauma systems, go wrong in only so many ways. Things fail along the same lines. Some examples are the identification of trauma patients, triage of the critically ill and injured, surgical decision-making, and surgeon arrival, including notification. When you do a FMEA analysis, you can imagine how things could go wrong, sometimes in ways people without the tool can't. You can see projects that aren't even on the radar for other people. That happens a lot, which is why FMEA is so useful. You can then explain to people, in an objective way, "We don't even know we have this problem because we can't detect it easily. Our systems don't even highlight that we have trouble with getting trauma patients to the OR because the surgeons frequently don't show in a timely fashion. The sick patient is dead long before any question of going to the OR comes up, so some of the other issues, such as time to the OR, go unrecognized in a system like ours."

STRATIFYING WITH FMEA

FMEA is most useful when it comes to big organizational goals. What are the big six things you've got to improve? You put them through the FMEA tool, and you can then stratify them. The highest risk score should get the top priority. Rigid adherence to the tool, however, can be counterproductive. Judgment is needed. The top-rated priority may not be achievable in the current circumstances. If you just can't do it, for whatever reason, you've got to take it off the list. The practicality dimension needs to be considered.

Organizations often can't have the hard conversations they need to have with themselves. If they're serious about quality improvement, they often need to bring in an objective outside consultant who can build some sort of consensus at the highest possible level, such as a steering committee, medical executive board, or board of directors. This is never easy, but when the consultant uses a neutral tool such as FMEA, the results are harder to argue with. When the consultant comes back to the leadership and says, "The tool shows this project is priority one," the question to ask the consultant next is "Is this doable?" The discussion at that point can usually be brief, because the executives know the organization better than the consultant does. The idea is that the consultant simply reports what the tool says, then facilitates using the tool as the basis of a discussion on what to do next. FMEA helps get the group's attention focused on the problems. It helps them prioritize and find a starting point instead of running in all directions.

Based on my experience, the initial FMEA presentation should be as high up on the organizational chart as you can get. Keep the presentations short—you don't usually get a lot of time, maybe only five or ten minutes. At the first meeting, get ideas for what projects they think are important and just list them. At the next meeting, arrive with suggested risk scores for each project. Ask the group for input and ask if they want to revise those numbers up and down. And remember, FMEA is only one dimension you can use to assess which project to do. Others include probability of success, how many resources the project will tie up, political/cultural limitations, and the potential COPQ you may recover.

From the time you first present to the group to the time you can get down to work on whatever quality-improvement project is approved can take four to six weeks or more. It's often useful to try to get it done in one or two meetings. The project itself may not get much, if any, budget. The timeline for early projects will usually be five to six months. Having a champion for the project, preferably someone in the hospital administration, is a big help for moving the project along and overcoming friction points. If there's no champion support for the team, the project isn't going to happen—at least not successfully.

PRACTICAL PROJECTS

Some projects are easier than others. Some make great projects for resident staff or any group with limited time and require only a very straightforward tool. One of the all-time greats for that sort of low-budget project, one that needs to be done quickly with low effort and maximal return, is the creation of a spaghetti diagram to discover wasted steps and wasted motion. In one project I supervised, we were able to cut an entire day and a half of walking out of the lives of ER nurses over a year. All it took was some simple redesign of the trauma resuscitation bays to move some things to better locations and to set things up better in advance. The nurses then didn't have to walk all over the floor to find what they needed. Also, now there weren't long periods where the patient was all alone. In fact, once the nurses didn't need to leave the room to get what they needed, we saw fewer self-extubations. These occur when patients cough out or remove their breathing tube, as sometimes happens when no one is present to redose them on sedation medication or otherwise intervene.

This sort of time-and-motion study is pretty routine in manufacturing and other areas. Medicine is late to the party, but we're getting there. We don't change things in medicine quickly, because safety is the top priority. Perhaps it's safer to change very slowly. (Of course, when there's a glaring issue, it's probably *less* safe to change slowly!) Also, health-care staff are busy (isn't everyone) with little to no time carved out for an improvement project. We're typically focused on seemingly more immediate issues. We'd rather stick with something that gives us what our gut tells us are pretty good outcomes, even if a rigorous look at the data (for the issue we don't have time for) would tell us that the defect rate is totally unacceptable in an important field that involves the health of human beings.

CHAPTER 3

JOHN KOTTER AND THE EIGHT STEPS OF CULTURE CHANGE

The hospital administrator had only been on the job for a few weeks, and he was already feeling frustrated. When he met the surgeon in the second floor café for their weekly chat about quality improvement, he barely greeted him before launching into a rant about how hard it was to get the tiniest little quality-improvement change to happen. He burst out, "I've just come from a meeting with the emergency-department people about trying to get incoming patients to the triage nurse a little sooner. One of the residents had a good idea about changing the intake form to make it easier to fill out. When I suggested doing that, though, all I heard were objections and complaints. I feel like they ganged up on me! If this is what happens with a change that's a no-brainer, what's going to happen when we get down to bigger projects?"

The surgeon sighed. "You've just had your first experience with butting up against the culture of an organization. What's going to happen going forward is that some good projects will fail because culture change is very, very hard to accomplish. But on the other hand, I've also seen that it can be done, if you use the right approach and have a thick skin."

+ + +

I've done a lot of quality projects at medical centers. The truth is, I'm good at them. I get brought in to medical centers as a consultant, and sometimes as an employee, to do quality turnarounds. Over the years, some projects worked out well; others weren't as successful as I had hoped; some were outright failures. All started as good, well-planned projects with clear objectives and a good road map for getting there. Yet something went wrong about 60 percent of the time. (That's a good batting average for the work I take on!) What I've learned from years of experience is that you can do all the Lean Six Sigma steps really well and in the right order, and the odds are still against you for culture change. It's very hard to modify a healthcare organization through innovation and invention. You have to do everything you can to ensure success and still be ready for failure. Let me share some personal advice for you if you consider walking the path of the change agent.

First, ask yourself if this is all worth it. I mean really think about it. Is what you're about to do worth it? The organization you're helping is the way it is for a reason. These are often deep reasons ingrained over *years* in ways you can't fathom when you start helping with the tools in this book. Will the outcome you can reasonably expect make this attempt (this "moment at bat" for culture change) worth your time and effort? I answer this question (commonly) with a yes. At the end of the organizational funnel are the patients, and if I see that there's a lot of good to be done for them, I've often said I'm in.

If you're going to embark on a path of culture change, if you're setting out to really make something different, you first have to be ready and resilient in yourself. You have to be mentally and emotionally prepared for the hits that are going to come at you. You have to be robust enough to deal with the ad hominem attacks that are an inevitable part of change. In healthcare, you can expect people to attack you rather than the changes you suggest. Some of the most vicious meetings I've ever been in were called because of something that wasn't a problem, but someone wanted to make a problem just to put an obstacle in the project's way (or sometimes just in your personal way).

In some cultures, change gets viewed as a fight. That's why reframing quality improvement in your organization as jointly collecting, processing, and *making changes based on data* is the key. There's no fight, because we just do what the data tell us to do! Beware the organization that doesn't let good data change its collective mind, whether that's because it can't collect data, buries data, attacks the people who want to use data, lacks the infrastructure to understand/process data, can't implement changes based on data, or can't maintain changes once made. I would submit that organizations that have a healthy approach to data-driven change are the ones poised to succeed when new challenges arise in the industry, such as the increasing focus on value of care over volume of service delivered. That's in direct contrast to organizations that view change as a personal fight or—perhaps just as bad—have no mechanism to adopt and implement only functional, useful changes.

Whatever the reasons that may happen in a particular place, it's no matter, because time will eventually wash such organizations away. Developing competency in each of those areas above is central to making sure we have an organization that responds as the playing field of health-care continues to change.

You can counteract some of the difficulties with culture change by being personally resilient and not taking anything personally, even when it's directed at you in a very personal manner. (Easy to say, tough to do!) You have to be resilient enough that when the earthworks are built and the battlements are created, and when people come at you, you're ready. You need to be better than good at all the basic things that are part of your daily life as a physician, administrator, or staff member, such as processing e-mails and signing off on documents, because there will be a lot of other demands on your time when resistance stresses your system.

You're the change agent, which means you're the lightning rod. Expect to be struck by lightning. Your tempo has to be quicker at many common tasks so that it isn't so easy to disrupt your decision loop. That doesn't mean you should rush through things; it just means you should get all your systems in place so that they can weather the storm. It's one thing to be able to guide the ship when the waters are calm. It's another thing when you have to steer it quickly and under duress when you're in the middle of a storm.

Now that my personal advice to you as a potential advocate

for quality is out there, let's take a look at some specific steps of culture change.

THE STEPS OF CULTURE CHANGE

John P. Kotter, a professor at the Harvard Business School, wrote a seminal article in 1995 called "Leading Change: Why Transformation Efforts Fail." It's the best, most definitive analysis I've ever seen of what needs to occur to make a culture change happen. In the article, Professor Kotter outlines eight crucial factors for success:

1. **Establish a sense of urgency.** Examine market and competitive realities; identify crises, potential crises, and major opportunities.

2. **Form a powerful guiding coalition.** Assemble a group with enough power to lead the change effort; encourage the group to work as a team.

3. **Create a vision.** A powerful vision helps direct the change effort. Develop strategies for achieving the vision.

4. **Communicate the vision.** Communicate the new vision and strategies every way you can. Teach new behaviors by the example of the guiding coalition.

5. **Empower others to act on the vision.** Get rid of obstacles to change; change systems and structures that seriously undermine the vision. Encourage risk-taking and nontraditional ideas, activities, and actions.

6. **Plan for and create short-term wins.** Plan for visible performance improvements, create them, and recognize and reward the people involved in the improvements.

7. **Consolidate improvements and produce still more change.** Use increased credibility from short-term wins to change systems, structures, and policies that don't fit the vision. Hire, promote, and develop employees who can implement the vision. Keep the process alive with new projects, themes, and change agents.

8. **Institutionalize new approaches.** Point out the connections between the new behaviors and corporate success. Develop ways to ensure leadership development and succession.

ESTABLISHING URGENCY

Organizations need a reason to change. It could be that a serious quality issue has come up, or maybe the hospital down the street has started a competing new service, and you're going to lose patients to them unless you start something similar. Whatever the reason for the change, if there's no sense of urgency, the change just won't happen in anything like a timely manner, or even at all.

I like to highlight the reason for the change and make sure everybody knows why it needs to be made. That gives it urgency and a sense of importance. A term that we sometimes use is the *burning platform*. The idea is to make people feel as if they're standing on a burning platform, so they have to do something fast to avoid being consumed by the flames. If you make everything into a burning platform, however, people will think you're an alarmist, and they'll completely shut off to you. You can't create a burning platform too often or for things that are inconsequential. When you do it, you've got to do it for something that really matters. I believe it should be used sparingly, only for big things.

At one hospital center where I worked, the administration didn't think they needed to do anything about the patient volume at their emergency department. They had a strong relationship with the local emergency medical services (EMS) providers. EMS routinely brought all their trauma patients to the hospital; everyone was happy with the arrangement. But then the big hospital down the road invested the money and work to become an accredited trauma center.

EMS has to follow a set of rules about where they bring injured patients. If the patient is anywhere near a designated trauma center, EMS has to bring them there, not to the nearest emergency department (ED). This has an influence on referral patterns, yet the hospital center didn't think it was important—or at least some parts of the hospital didn't. Perhaps they didn't see themselves aligned with the hospital as a whole for some reason. The team trying to do culture change at the hospital tried to create a sense of urgency about the upcoming shift in the ED patient mix, but they couldn't manage it. Important portions of the hospital didn't support the trauma center initiative going on in their own center, didn't communicate with the EMS providers, and didn't do anything to improve its own ability to handle serious trauma. Not surprisingly, the hospital center's ED lost 15 percent of its visits over the next year and a half once a trauma center opened down the road. This really hurt the hospital's bottom line, to the point where it went into a decline that couldn't be halted. The hospital eventually closed.

A trauma center brings a lot more to a hospital than just life-saving skills for seriously injured patients. The trauma center increases patient volume, but it also improves the hospital's ability to care for critically ill and injured patients. It also allows a center to handle big surgical procedures that might even need things such as expanded blood bank services to help rescue patients who have problems in the OR.

Trauma elevates all ships in the bay, but there's a problem: from an accounting standpoint, a hospital often doesn't know what trauma patients bring to it until they're not coming there anymore. The opposite can happen as well. This is why I share this example: the culture change steps (and tools like the COPQ) can often reframe how a hospital thinks of certain service lines such as trauma and acute-care surgery. Without care, a hospital can, for a variety of reasons, lose its designation as a trauma center. Trauma patients get taken elsewhere. And because the emergency department is an important outward-facing part of the hospital, the loss of the trauma center means the community eventually has less confidence in the ED and uses it less, often preferring to go to the hospital that does have a trauma center or simply being forced to go to another nearby hospital ED because of regulations that EMS must follow.

All this requires Kotter's eight steps when a group tries to avoid this outcome and to focus on value delivered to people in the local community.

FORMING A POWERFUL GUIDING COALITION

Institutional support is crucial for cultural change. When

this support comes in the form of a group made up of individuals with enough power to lead the change effort and also willing to work together, the change is lot more likely to happen and to stick. The group not only needs to have an interest in making the change; it also needs to contain people who have the authority to make changes. This is the group that will be able to influence the staff and the hospital administration and help them move in the direction they need to go. You've got to build a group of people who are going to take it there. Things are the way they are at a hospital center for a reason. To make changes, the group has to be consciously willing to push through all the forces that are aligned against it.

Do not take a culture change role if your potential superiors don't have the patience, political savvy, and just plain strong stomach that it takes for culture change. This doesn't mean that you plan to "run wild" and expect carte blanche support because you're the lightning rod. I'm telling you that any pushback you get will be in the form of bad reports via things like poisonous letters written about you. That's what pushback looks like, even when you treat people right. Sometimes the bad report will even go over the head of your boss in an attempt to manipulate or subvert the improvement process.

I've seen it all in healthcare. Be ready. Form a strong

guiding coalition, and don't accept a role in a turnaround where there's not a strong guiding coalition in place or one that's *very* easy to make.

CREATING A VISION

Once the group is assembled, you have to work together to make the form of the strategic vision very clear to them. You won't be able to communicate that vision if it's not clear and direct. I like to get the vision down to one very clear sentence, an ultrashort pitch that lays out the vision and where it needs to go. Remember, some of the group members are your bosses, and so really they're setting the preconditions for change.

COMMUNICATING THE VISION

The members of the change group have to be willing, even eager, to participate. They have to sign on to the strategic vision and be willing to take the hits that can come with that. They have to be willing to lead by example. The change group is sometimes compared to a volunteer army—they volunteer to be in the line of fire instead of waiting to be drafted. What makes the change group work is that they all share the vision and really want to see the project succeed. They're your ambassadors to the rest of the organization for communicating the vision.

To empower others to act, barriers have to be removed in any way you can. This is where calculated risk-taking and creative thinking can be very helpful. Barriers to change are typically processes or structures that have evolved to favor the older, less functional way of doing things. The truth is, health-care systems aren't good or bad. They're either functional or dysfunctional, yet people in healthcare have trouble seeing it that way. We have a lot of trouble getting past judging the individuals and seeing just the function. The question to ask is, "Is this system functional for what you now need, or not?" If it isn't, changes have to be made, and that usually means removing and changing processes—and sometimes people—that favor how things are (the current state), instead of how they need to be for the system to improve. In many places throughout healthcare, it seems to be particularly difficult to avoid personalizing changes.

The barriers need to fall, but that's very difficult. People get comfortable with things the way they are, even if the system isn't working very well and ways to improve are obvious. It's very hard to make people work in an uncomfortable way. That said, I advise doing everything possible to engage the people who are on the ground already when the change effort starts. Show clearly what is expected to happen if the organization doesn't improve the value it delivers. Help them imagine how that affects them and everyone. Ask them to help with specific changes (including that data-driven approach) that can help avoid the pain and consequence of not acting differently.

In fact, one of the most difficult barriers to change in healthcare may include people who stand in the way of the vision in ways they sometimes don't even realize. Unfortunately, that sometimes means you have to transition some people out. (That's my least favorite option, but it's necessary sometimes.) Remember, there are reasons why an organization that needs substantial change is how it is: prior history, current staff—these and lots of reasons conspire to keep things how they are.

PLAN FOR SHORT-TERM WINS

Planning for early wins is key for getting a change to stick. As soon as you possibly can, show that your new process or system is doing something good. Highlight the heck out of it. Talk it up constantly at internal meetings. You need to do this to encourage the change team and the people they're working with and to counteract the naysayers. In the same meeting where you report a solid short-term gain, they will invariably complain about some aspect of your new process or system or point out some shortcoming (usually in you, but sometimes in the project such as a downside to the change). You need to be prepared for this response and not get discouraged about exposing yourself to attack every time you report a small step forward.

As you plan your quality-improvement project, ask yourself, "Where am I going to see early wins? What can I measure to show success quickly?" You have to have something that the team and everyone else can feel and notice. Look for a goal or endpoint that's as visible and tangible as possible, and find a way to achieve it early on.

If it's appropriate, talk with the public-relations people at the hospital. A positive article in the local paper does a lot to build credibility for the project. Most health centers are too big for the PR department to bother with a small internal success, however. I focus on internal marketing just by telling everyone I can as often as I can about anything good, while complimenting and rewarding the people involved as much as I can.

CONSOLIDATE IMPROVEMENTS AND PRODUCE MORE CHANGE

Once you get the changes going, lean in. Start to speed up the pace of change. When you feel that things are reaching a tipping point, when you sense a barrier is about to fall, when you think something's about to give, push it as far as you can and as fast as you can. Once you get a couple of early wins, that means things are going in your favor, and they're building on themselves. Now's the time to push hard for even faster change. Push even at the risk of going a little too far. Try to get the system to look like the ideal you're aiming for. Do it, because eventually things will pull back from the ideal and settle down somewhere around a less-than-perfect but more acceptable and sustainable endpoint.

INSTITUTIONALIZE NEW APPROACHES

Making an ongoing difference with your quality changes is the final and most important step. Make sure the rest of the administration sees that the changes you've made are not only improving quality in whatever department you're in but also improving the center overall. When you can show better patient outcomes, cost savings, reduced staff turnover, and all the other things that the organization really cares about, you'll get the institutional support that helps make the changes stick. At the same time, you need to build support from the bottom up. Bring in people who will deploy and improve the new process or system; if you must, let go of the people who obstruct it.

Be sure that the system you want to put in place is a good one. Even if you have everybody on board and have followed all the steps for success, if the system is so bad that it fails right from the start, you're not going to want to keep it going. Cut your losses, because a bad system empowers the people who push back against change.

THE IMPORTANCE OF CULTURE CHANGE

When you're working within a health-care system, it's sometimes very difficult to see the bigger picture and acknowledge that there's a lot of room for improvement. We always want to think we're doing well. We always want to think we're doing the best we can and working hard, which is almost always the case. Very few people in healthcare say, "Look, I know I'm lazy. I know I'm really not doing a very good job. Meh. Who cares?" Nobody does that, because people go into healthcare because they do care. The problem in culture change is the problem of looking at the data—standing back and looking at the whole system. That's why following the culture change steps in sequence is important. You need to establish an urgency people can feel. Without that sense of urgency and ability to create change, people will say, "Why would I want to put in the work to fix this? It's not worth it."

To get past that and build enthusiasm for change, people have to be willing to follow you and spend the time on the project. What influences people to follow someone or make changes isn't always what you think. You could have the best data in the world showing that a change is necessary, and that still won't influence people to follow you. In fact, it typically doesn't, because data can't overcome the emotional and sometimes financial investment people have in a situation.

Many, many books have been written about what gets people to follow or change. I've read a lot of them, and in my view, there are many good points to be had. I feel that if you want to improve your leadership and get people to follow you, there's no one expert who has all the answers. Look at the leading titles, read them through, and pick the leadership model you feel most comfortable with. Just go with it. Personally, I like the cognitive elaboration model, which builds on prior knowledge to form associations with new information. I find my personal style of leadership is more like whispering in someone's ear than grabbing him by the nose and pulling him along. With rare exceptions, I don't like to tell people exactly what to do.

Leading by example is often said to be the most effective approach, but it's hard to do in healthcare. Everybody's working so hard that sometimes you wonder if they notice that you're setting an example. They don't notice that you came in at two in the morning, because everybody does that. What works best for me is coaching people, mentoring them, and bringing them along.

IMPROVING THE ODDS

Realistically speaking, the odds of a new quality initiative succeeding are relatively low, only about 40 percent. What can you do to improve your chance of success? Aside from getting your life aligned so that you can devote the right level of energy and persistence to the project, try to create something viral.

I like to use ideas that are sticky—they're easy to grasp, and they resonate with people both intellectually and emotionally. When I'm making the case for the project and keeping people motivated as it moves forward, I try to tell a compelling story. I like to use selected patient cases that will show what the problem is and how the new system will fix it in human terms. Stories resonate with people more than data charts. I love the data more than anything, but it's not the influencer for most people. They don't understand it and don't want to be bothered to know what it means. They're much more responsive to things that are visceral and memorable. If you package the project with a good story, it makes a big difference.

OVERCOMING ROADBLOCKS

When—not if—you run into roadblocks trying to follow Kotter's eight steps, don't panic. Roadblocks are expected in this process. Step back and reassess. Review the steps so far to see if they're in place and working OK. If not, go back and make corrections. You may need to change around your guiding coalition to make sure everyone on it is looking out for you and being supportive, not just sitting quietly in the background or being a bystander. If you're not getting full cooperation, go back to the group and make the case again to create that sense of urgency. Are you sure they get what you're talking about? Are they seeing it only through the lens of their job titles, whether as finance director or medical director or any other job title? What makes something urgent to them?

I've found that asking the guiding coalition to imagine various scenarios is helpful for creating urgency. How would it look if we lost a patient because we didn't do this quality project? If you would lose a patient, then it's such a catastrophic possibility that you've got to act.

Sometimes you just have to go to someone on the coalition and ask him or her to be more vocal. That team member is on board but is being too quiet. People do sometimes need to be encouraged. Your coalition members are busy people with a lot of responsibilities and distractions, especially if the organization has a high administrative burden. They have a lot of issues to deal with every day. They believe in the quality project and are glad they're on the team, but to them it's also just one more thing, not *the* thing. What makes this thing stand out? To keep them engaged and supportive, you have to answer that important question for them.

PEOPLE, NOT MATH

Lean Six Sigma is a type of programmed culture change. Through its steps, it automatically does many of the changes Kotter suggests, in that order. They're hardwired into the process.

When people first learn Lean Six Sigma, they tend to think it's all math and statistics. In reality, we always say it's 80 percent people and 20 percent math. It's a specific version, in many ways, of Kotter's eight culture-change steps. It's mostly about the people and the setup. The 20 percent that's math is vital, but it's not the main thing. If you don't have good people skills and aren't interested in the culture change, being able to do the math isn't going to help you.

Of course, you can have great people skills and great math skills and still get struck by lightning during your quality-improvement project. It pays to have a big toolbox and be willing to use everything in it to get the project done. Sometimes you even have to be willing to be hard on people, although I recommend that tool be used the least. That should be the tool that's the shiniest in your toolbox, because you use it so rarely.

CHAPTER 4

THE STAKEHOLDERS AND THE DATA: DMAIC

When the hospital administrator next joined the surgeon for their weekly coffee meeting, he found the surgeon shuffling through a pile of paper and scribbling on a notepad.

"What's all that?"

The surgeon answered, "I'm working on the project charter for that quality-improvement project on avoiding medication delays. We had a lot of stakeholders in the room, so I have to incorporate a lot of perspectives to get the charter worded right."

The administrator replied, "Actually, I have a meeting like that in a couple of days. We're going to talk about improving the time from admission in the ED to actually getting the patient into a bed upstairs. The ED people gave me a list of stakeholders. They acted all surprised when I asked them to include someone from the patient-transport team on it."

"Good call about that," the surgeon said. "Step one is always to get everyone in the room. Only then can you move on to the DMAIC steps."

"I sort of remember that D-whatever stuff from my MBA. Do we really have to work through all those steps? It seems as if it'll add a lot of time to the planning."

"Never, ever skip DMAIC," said the surgeon. "The time you spend now thinking through every step of the project will save you tons of time later on."

+ + +

In one organization, when a patient is scheduled for surgery, a surgical booker (also called a surgical coordinator) is the person who handles all the details, such as insurance coverage and making sure all the presurgical steps are done. At one hospital where I worked, the administration decided to do a quality-improvement program for the surgery department. They had grand designs for how to reorganize the department, including changing what the bookers would do and how they did it. The only problem was that they never asked the bookers if they thought the changes were good ideas. A month after the program was implemented, only one of the original bookers was still working there. The others quit.

One of the most important things for a successful quality-improvement project is making sure the stakeholders who will be affected are in the room. Only they really understand the process you want to improve.

STARTING OUT WITH DMAIC

In Lean Six Sigma, the acronym DMAIC (pronounced "dah may ick") is used to mean the steps of the process-improvement system: define, measure, analyze, improve, control. Each aspect is a step on the path toward improving the process. Checkpoints called tollgates are used to make sure each step has been completed before moving on to the next.

DEFINE: THE PROJECT CHARTER

Step one is to define. In this step, you define the project by creating a project charter—the tool that defines the scope of the project, who the stakeholders are, the timeline for completion, and the expected cost savings in terms of the cost of poor quality.

When you do the stakeholder analysis for this first step, you've got to get the people who participate in the process in the room. You can't know what the project is really about unless they're there to provide their input. You have to consider all the stakeholders, even the ones you may intuitively think don't need to be there. They might actually need to be there. In the case of the surgical bookers, for instance, they weren't included because the focus was on OR use. The bookers were seen as just the people who did the paperwork, but in fact, they were key to getting patients onto the OR schedule. When you map any quality-improvement process out, a lot of people are involved. In the search for solutions, you've got to get them in the room. You can't sign people up for things if they're not part of the process.

The downside of including all the stakeholders can be really big, unwieldy meetings. Too many stakeholders means you can't get anywhere. When you make the process map, all the people who have a legitimate stake in it need to be included. You need to use your judgment about who to ask, however, because the group also needs to be manageable. The project leader or Lean Six Sigma black belt usually has a good sense of who the main players are.

Once the project charter has been defined, the next toll-gate is to come up with a SIPOC diagram. SIPOC stands for suppliers, input, process, output, and customers. This diagram is developed with input from everyone in the group. A good approach is to start in the middle with the process column and develop around five or six steps that define it at a very high level. In healthcare, we typically tend to be overly detailed about process, but really, experience shows that five to six high-level steps will suffice.

Once the group agrees on what the process is, then they come up with the rest of the information.

One important aspect of this process—perhaps the most important part—is called the Voice of the Customer (VOC), meaning customer needs and requirements. This is where Lean Six Sigma can get very challenging in healthcare, because it's not always clear who the customer is. Is it the patient receiving the care? Is it the third-party insurer who reimburses the health system? Is it both? Sometimes the VOC is a state regulatory body or an accrediting agency. The VOC is a good way to define what a defect is. If the state regulatory agency says that a trauma surgeon has to be at the trauma bay within fifteen minutes of patient arrival, that's the definition. Anything longer than fifteen minutes is a defect.

Do you see the issue? Who gets to define what *valuable* is when we work on going from volume of services delivered to value of services delivered? Choosing the VOC carefully for a particular project is an essential part of improving the value we deliver in healthcare.

By contrast, for health-care projects, the inputs are often much more clear than they are in other businesses. In many health-care projects, the major input is the patient. The suppliers are more varied. For example, a patient needs a back brace. The suppliers would then be the brace manufacturer, the specialist who determined that a brace is necessary, and the emergency department or floor nurse who supplies the brace to the patient. Often, for trauma-type SIPOC diagrams, EMS is a key supplier.

Next, it's time to determine the output. The output is often the patient, with some additional feature or value added, such as the patient with a back brace.

Finally, we come to the customers. This is where things may also get challenging, because it can be very difficult to determine who the customer is in healthcare. The customer may be a third-party payer, the patient, other physicians, EMS, or the trauma service. It may be the back-brace patient and also the social worker who does his discharge planning. The physical therapist and occupational therapy team may also be customers. Of course, physical therapy and occupational therapy may also be suppliers, because their evaluations and recommendations are part of the decision to give the patient a back brace and send him for physical and occupational therapy. The bottom line is that we have to identify clearly who the customers are in our health-care quality-improvement project so that the VOC we take is the applicable one.

Clearly, completion of a SIPOC diagram is essential. If you don't do this step, you'll have a difficult time deciding what to measure to focus the project and achieve success.

MEASURE: COLLECTING THE DATA AND GENERATING ENDPOINTS

The information you've gathered in the SIPOC phase lets you move on to the measurement phase. The group uses the SIPOC information to select which parameters to measure to characterize the system. The information is also used to help the team generate and agree on meaningful endpoints.

In the measure phase, a data-collection plan is created. The data-collection plan includes what measures you think have validity and should be measured. The number of things to measure should be large enough to detect changes in the system and be statistically valid. At the same time, the number of data points doesn't have to be large. Often only two input measures and two output measures are enough. The Lean Six Sigma black belt can help the group choose the right things to measure and figure out what the correct sample size should be. This step is very important, because you need to establish a baseline sigma level to know how the system is currently performing. That value helps tell you about how much variation there is in the process you're looking at.

Everybody in the group gets to help define what the outcome measures mean. This is really important, because you need to build consensus around the data you're going to get. The process is very methodical—you do all the defining and decision-making before you go out and measure anything.

The measurement step depends on whether the group gets a valid sample. We try to avoid data from data warehouses or retrospective data from databases. Ideally, we want to get clean data prospectively from the site, from the actual process itself, rather than getting it later from the computer or looking at retrospective data from a log. That's really key. If we're measuring how long it takes for patients coming in to the ED to see the triage nurse, for instance, we want to have someone on the spot with a clipboard and a stopwatch. Retrospective reports tend to be very beautiful and clean, but not accurate.

Sample size is an important consideration. How big does the sample size need to be in order to be useful? It depends on how big a magnitude of change you want to be able to detect. Let's say you want the smallest change you can detect to be a 40 percent change. A 40 percent change is pretty nongranular, so in that case, you'd be able to detect change in a smaller sample. If you wanted to make the smallest detectable change be a 1 percent change, you would need a lot more data, which means a much bigger sample size. The Lean Six Sigma black belt running the data collection can use the right equations to figure out the sample size you need. (You can find the equations on my website at http://bit.ly/1IAgpTi.)

Once you know how big your sample needs to be, you have a pretty good idea of how long it's going to take to gather the data. You probably already know how many patients pass through the system, so you have a sense of how many are relevant to your study. Knowing how long it will take to get the data is useful, because you don't want to make changes along the way until you have a valid sample. You have to wait until you've completed your data collection to make any changes. That prevents tampering—that is, making a change and then making another change right away. Tampering only confuses the bigger picture and can make things worse, so you want to avoid it (see chapter 9 for more on this). Wait until you have a valid sample set to see the outcome.

People have a tendency to put analysis ahead of the data. They'll start throwing out solutions long before the data comes in. Everybody thinks he or she knows the answer, because we live in the system and we feel we know its flaws from personal experience. Often, we're right, but not always. And "not always" makes a big difference.

You really want to make sure you have data and measurements before you go with what your gut tells you is going to work. You have to have some data before you put a solution in. The data will validate—or not—what people think the solution ought to be.

ANALYZE: STATISTICAL TESTING AND DATA EVALUATION

Sometimes the data gives you an unexpected or counterintuitive answer. That's the power of data: the power to change your mind, because you can't argue with the numbers. In one project I worked on, the data told us there was a problem in the computer system with the autotext that generated a physician's daily progress note. We thought we knew why our coders were telling us that we couldn't bill for certain encounters, and it turns out we were completely incorrect. Collecting and using data according to this pathway allowed us to scramble less to see more patients (volume) and to make a correction that allowed us to document the value we were already providing. It made a difference of $200,000 per year, and it was all because we took our cues from data rather than from what our gut told us was wrong.

The Lean Six Sigma black belt does the data analysis and the statistical testing. The statistical testing is done after the improvements have been made to see how well they're doing. The data analysis can take a long time. In my experience, after all the work that went into defining the project, gathering the data, and then analyzing it, the meeting to present the results of the analysis only takes about an hour. The black belt presents the data to the group and explains how to visualize and interpret it. The group usually understands right away how well the quality-improvement project is performing. If it's doing well or if it's doing badly, the data will tell you exactly. It's inarguable, because the group has agreed in advance about what the endpoints are.

The great beauty of this approach is that nobody feels as if it's a hunt for the guilty. That's very powerful. The Lean Six Sigma process places a cross-disciplinary team on the same page. The process makes the current state of performance very clear to everyone without being pejorative. It shows the business case for why change is worthwhile. It points out where our everyday experience of the system doesn't line up with the data. The statistics reveal places where we think we're doing well but really aren't. They change our minds about the way forward.

If the data tell us the program isn't working, we then have to talk about what to do to fix it. This can be very challenging. An approach I like to use is to say, "Go to the literature and find solutions that other people have done. Or ask friends at other hospitals what they've done. Bring those ideas with you to the next meeting, and we'll talk about them." At the next meeting, we select the ideas we think would work well and can be done here. Usually it takes one or two meetings to get everybody's head wrapped around what does and doesn't work. It's an iterative process.

When we first work on a healthcare process, we typically find a defect rate that's about equal to what's seen in any service industry before a quality-improvement initiative. That's about one defect for every one thousand opportunities. In healthcare, that rate would mean defects are rare and barely noticeable on a day-to-day basis. That makes it acceptable, in part because (I think) it's difficult to feel. In other areas, that level would be unacceptably high. In air travel, for instance, one defect per thousand would mean a plane crashing every day at every busy airport.

Typically, when I teach courses in Lean Six Sigma, I share that a 4.5 sigma level (one defect in around 250,000 opportunities) is achievable with an excellent program. To get to a higher sigma level in healthcare (or any industry) often requires a complete overhaul of the system. (We call that the "engine transplant.") The radical ideas that are needed to do that are very difficult to achieve.

So, when someone proposes a radical change, I usually take the time to embrace it by thinking about it with the team during a meeting. That's because such ideas are rarely seen; and, although most don't come to fruition, the ones that do are often the only ones that hold potential to get beyond 4.5 sigma. I say, "OK, if we're going to go this route, this is a major overhaul. This takes time, money, and commitment." At the same time, you have to tell the group, "A good solution has to be implementable. Are we going to go for the home run with this, or are we going to go for the iterative change?" I leave that decision up to the group. Usually, perhaps unfortunately, organizations are not ready or able to run with the ideas that can get us to the value seen beyond 4.5 sigma. But maybe one day they will.

Some things can't be achieved, because they cost too much or they're prohibitive in some other way, such as needing too much staff. We usually end up tabling these ideas for later. That's a shame, because it's possible that those radical ideas could either fail fabulously or be the home runs that revolutionize the system. Unfortunately, we rarely end up knowing. We're just looking for iterative improvements. We often choose incremental over radical.

IMPROVE: FINDING INNOVATIVE SOLUTIONS

The next step after analysis is to improve. The *improve* phase has several tollgates, including stakeholder-generated solutions. Once the data has been analyzed and shared, the stakeholders can generate new and different solutions or think of ways to improve the solution. Then the same selection process as earlier is applied: How easily can the solution be implemented? What resources will it take? How will it impact the system? The new solutions are implemented, and the data is collected again and analyzed. Because you've already made changes using this process, you already have the structure for getting the data, so it goes more smoothly.

This time, the data analysis focuses on how the system looks now. The group has to be very honest this time, as honest as they were in the first iteration. Again, that's very challenging, because you often need to reassure them, "You're not going to get fired for this. It's not a witch hunt; we're not looking to say who's bad. It's not personal. It's just data."

Once a system has been improved, the control phase is set up to do an ongoing review of it. That way, if it goes awry, you'll be able to know quickly. The control phase is one of the toughest, because you have to set it up so that it keeps the momentum going even when you're not looking in on it. Projects that do succeed in changing outcomes often fall off, meaning they don't maintain their improvement. A response plan is generated so that when the system sends a signal that it's having quality issues, we know what to do.

A range of Lean Six Sigma tools for the review process tell us when to check back on the system or resample the data. In healthcare, one of the most effective tools is a control chart called the individuals and moving range (I-MR) chart. This works well, because patients come through the system one at a time. Tools such as control charts are effective, but you really need an expert in data to show you how to use them. That's because understanding these charts requires a good grasp of the underlying math. I-MR charts can be particularly misleading if you don't have expertise. These charts, for example, typically assume data are normally distributed, but sometimes the data you've gotten from the system doesn't have a normal distribution. This can be seriously misleading if you don't adjust for it. I see control charts being used incorrectly in healthcare all the time.

To give just one example, at one hospital I helped, we had an issue with the surgeons supervising residents. We had built and validated our own scale about how well the attending surgeons supervised resident surgeons. We had a way to demonstrate that we were supervising them well. We had developed a continuous data endpoint. We got to be pretty good at using the scale. We showed statistically significant improvement, and the system felt better. Plus, we just knew we were doing a better job. When we went to set up the control phase, it turned out we couldn't use a routine I-MR chart, because it would mislead us to think that everything was OK even if things weren't OK. We would have to handle our data differently when we set up the control phase. It was all because our data didn't follow the normal distribution.

Nonnormal data can handled by at least two options. One is to do a data transformation that will raise the data to a certain power. The Box-Cox transformation, for example, is often used to attempt to make nonnormal data into a normal distribution. For example, if the variable time isn't normally distributed, the Box-Cox transformation will take time and raise it to whatever power it takes to make the data become that typical normal curve that we all love. Of course, if the variable time had to be cubed to make it into a normal curve, what does that mean? Regardless, once you have the data transformed to normal distribution, you can then use typical control charts that assume a normal distribution. Knowing whether your data are normal or nonnormal, and what to do with each, is important. E-mail me if you have questions about how any tools or steps work with nonnormal data.

In the case of the surgeon supervision, we were in the control phase, still with a nonnormal data distribution. One of my colleagues put a control chart on the data one day and said, "Oh my gosh. This is terrible. We can't continue doing this. We've slipped way back. These two cases demonstrate we didn't supervise the resident adequately." I said, "Wait a minute. Look. Our original distribution was nonnormal." He hadn't performed a data transform to obtain a normal distribution and was led astray into thinking we had a problem that needed fixing. In fact, there really wasn't any unexpected variation, and the program was still working well. The correct answer from the control chart was that it was all fine, and we didn't have to make any changes.

Lean Six Sigma strongly encourages a learning attitude, so when I clarified why we really didn't have a problem, everyone was very collegial about it. They didn't take offense or argue; they said, "Oh, now I see it. We're good." Problem avoided. The best part was that the discussion completely centered around data and in no way was personal. We didn't even need to waste time looking at cases that weren't an issue!

DOES IT WORK?

Of the more than fifty major quality-improvement projects I've led, I've seen meaningful, statistically significant improvement in probably thirty-five of them. The projects were of varying degrees of importance and difficulty, so they can't be exactly compared. At least five made truly revolutionary improvements in value delivered to patients. The ones that didn't work were mostly clustered at one center that was very resistant to the data-driven way of making decisions. There's an old saying, "Culture eats strategy for breakfast." I can sort of understand that. Not everybody wants to (or can) shake things up, even if it's obviously for the better.

Entrenched culture can be hard to change. Again, the philosophy of wanting to improve with data is a necessary precursor for quality-improvement projects. That desire has to be there, or the project often doesn't get off the ground.

For process improvement, nothing works like Lean Six Sigma. Nothing. Statistical process control makes you look your performance square in the eye in a way that everybody agrees on. This process makes everyone agree on what the numbers mean and where the numbers say they should go.

CHAPTER 5

ABANDON YOUR INTUITION: COUNTERINTUITIVE SOLUTIONS SOMETIMES WORK

The hospital administrator arrived at the little second-floor café a few minutes late for his usual coffee meeting with the surgeon. "Sorry," he said. "I was in this long meeting trying to analyze a problem in the pathology lab. We just can't seem to get to the bottom of what's causing it."

The surgeon replied, "You know, there's a Lean Six Sigma tool for that."

"Why am I not surprised to hear that from you?" said the administrator. "What is it? I really need to know before I meet with those guys again."

"It's called the Five Whys. You act sort of like a four-year-old and just keep asking why something is. By the time you get to the fifth Why, you've usually managed to get to the root issue. What helps with this approach is that it doesn't need any math, so people are usually pretty open to trying it."

✢ ✢ ✢

When something bad happens in surgery, your experience of time seems to speed up. I worked with a surgeon who unexpectedly needed to give his patient fresh frozen plasma (FFP) during an operation. FFP takes about thirty minutes to thaw. The surgeon complained to me afterward, saying, "It took forever to get the FFP to me. We really need to completely change the system for delivering it to the OR." As the head of quality, I took his complaint seriously. The hospital's standard time requirement for delivering FFP is thirty minutes. In this case, the delivery took longer than that. Was this an outlier or a sign of a real problem? I wasn't sure, so I decided to check into the situation further. For the next one hundred FFP doses, we started the clock when the order went in, and we stopped it when the bag showed up at the patient's bedside. It turned out that we were actually doing pretty well with FFP dosing. There wasn't a lot of variation in the time it took to get the dose to the patient; almost all got there in just about thirty minutes. When we drilled down, we found that any delays were almost always caused by delays in putting in the order to begin with. The data clearly showed the system wasn't a terrible system. A few simple tweaks fixed the whole thing, but they weren't intuitive tweaks based on the one really tough situation that one surgeon had faced. When something goes wrong in a system, even if it seems to be just an outlier event and maybe not an underlying problem, checking into it can still be revealing. Your experience may tell you that a simple fix is all you need, but until you have data, you can't know that for sure. When you're at a patient's bedside, it's sometimes hard to see what's really conspiring to slow down your FFP delivery. Making changes without data usually just introduces more variation and has a lot of potential for making things worse.

That's what is so powerful about Lean Six Sigma techniques. We all have visceral reactions to bad outcomes. Lean Six Sigma takes the emotion out of the discussion. It makes us really look at making changes based on information, not intuition. Intuition can be a valuable guide, but intuition doesn't get you where you really want to go. Evolution has built our brains to make connections. Lightning strikes a log, the log bursts into flame, so we connect lightning with starting a fire. In reality, that's very rare. Lightning strikes all the time, and nothing catches fire. The one time it does, however, is what we remember. That's not systems-level thinking. Data-driven improvement works when you look at the complete picture of what the system really is, including the variations in it. You try to eliminate variation. You look at an event within the system, not just as something you've experienced, but as it fits in the bigger context.

SOLVING A BOTTLENECK

At one hospital where I worked, a problem with admission delays in the emergency department led us far astray when we tried to solve it intuitively. In fact, we made the situation worse. Patients were spending too much time in the emergency room after the decision to admit them was made. There was a lot of consternation about why it took so long and why we were routinely running over the hospital guidelines for admission. We had a lot of case-by-case discussion, trying to pinpoint where the bottleneck was. Finally, we decided to stop discussing and start gathering data. We did a prospective study and had one of the residents walk through the system. What we discovered was that a twenty-minute computer delay was built into the system. The doctor would get into the computer system and admit the patient, but the software took twenty minutes to tell the patient-transport staff that it was time to wheel the patient upstairs. That was a completely unexpected answer. We had been sitting around in meetings trying to figure out why the admission process took too long. We were saying things like, "This particular doctor didn't make a decision in a timely fashion." Sometimes that was actually true, but not always. It took using statistical tools to uncover what the real issue was.

We went to the information-technology (IT) people and showed them the data. We asked what we could do to help them fix the problem. By taking this approach, instead of blaming them for creating the problem, we turned them into stakeholders. They were able to fix the software issue, and we were able to shave twenty minutes off everyone's time in the ER. Looking back, we should probably have involved the IT department from the start.

Interestingly, by fixing a computer problem in one area, you sometimes end up fixing it elsewhere as well. That wasn't your original intent—you just wanted to get your own problem fixed—but sometimes you end up raising all the boats.

THE FIVE WHYS

Another Lean Six Sigma technique that works for revealing underlying problems is called the Five Whys. It's usually applied in the *analyze* phase of DMAIC as a way to get at a root cause. You keep asking why a problem is happening until you've drilled down to the real reason. You can almost always get there by the fifth Why. The fun part of the Five Whys is that, unlike a lot of other Lean Six Sigma tools, no statistical analysis is needed. Just get your group together and start asking, why? After you've asked the question five times, and you stop getting a different answer each time, you've gotten to the root causation.

In the case of the ER admission delay, the first why question was "Why is it taking us more than two hours to get patients out of the ED or admitted in general?" The answer was "It's taking us two hours because we call for transport, but transport's not available." "Why is transport not available?" "They're mostly busy with patients in the intensive-care unit." "Why are they mostly busy there?" "Because staffing is such that we don't have enough people." "Why are we understaffed?" "Because the budget was cut." Now we had reached the root cause— there were not enough patient-transport aides because the budget for them had been cut.

ISHIKAWA DIAGRAMS

Another Lean Six Sigma approach to root causes is an Ishikawa diagram, named for Kaoru Ishikawa, a Japanese organizational theorist who developed the idea in the 1960s. Based on the way it looks, an Ishikawa diagram is also called a fishbone diagram. The Ishikawa diagram helps you identify the factors you think correlate with a certain outcome—in other words, it identifies causes and effects. Among your group, there will often be differences of opinion about the root cause of a problem. At the same time, there may not be a lot of data. The value of the fishbone diagram is that it lets you visualize all the possible causes of a specific problem or effect. Or, to put it in Lean Six Sigma terms, the fishbone diagram highlights the multiple causes for a special cause variation—a variation above and beyond the normal variation expected in the system.

A special cause variation can almost always be traced to one of six categories: the "five Ms and one P," or materials, machine, method, mother nature, management, and people.

I used this approach to solve a problem we were having with delays in bringing on new physicians at my hospital. The delays were causing real problems, so we wanted to find out what was causing them and brainstorm a fast fix.

Once we started looking at the problem, we saw there were a lot of factors involved. We drew a horizontal line (the backbone of the fish) on the whiteboard, with the word *effect* all the way to the right (the head of the fish). For each of the five Ms and one P that we thought were important, we drew a vertical line out from the backbone (the bones of the fish).

Once we felt we had a good handle on the possible causes, we collected data prospectively on the next providers the hospital hired. We needed to find out if the factors we thought were associated with the delays really were. All a fishbone diagram really represents is what factors the group *thinks* are associated with the special cause variation. Until there's data, the fishbone diagram just represents opinions.

How can you make a fishbone diagram actionable? It needs to be combined with a multiple-regression model to turn it into a conclusion that will lead to tangible improvement. The factors you think are important need to be labeled as "controllable" or "noise." Said differently, we try to get a sense of which factors we have control over and which we don't. For example, we can't control the weather. If bad weather keeps the hiring committee from meeting, that can't be changed. Depending on how well the model fits the data, we may decide to see what happens if the elements that are beyond our control are removed from the model, leaving only the controllable elements. Next, we try to identify which fishbone elements are ones for which we have useful data already and which need to be collected. If we need more data, we then establish the usual sort of collection plan.

Once all the data is in place, we create a multiple-regression model using software such as Minitab. Getting a useful result may take some work—leave this part to your Lean Six Sigma black belt. In the end, when we get the multiple regression output, we look for an R^2 value that's greater than 0.80. An R^2 value of 0 would mean the model doesn't explain any of the variability. An R^2 value of 0.80 means that 80 percent of the variability in our outcome data is explained by the factors in the model. The higher the R^2 value, the better. Now we know the answer to the question "What portion of the variability in the outcome data is in our control based on choices we can make?" (Actually, we tend to use something called the R^2 adjusted, which is a bit stricter criterion to make sure the model is useful.)

As often happens, it turned out that many of the things we thought correlated with the delay didn't seem to reach significance. Working to improve those factors might not influence the time until the new physician got to work. We could see from the regression analysis that we needed to focus on ways to decrease the time from when a job application was submitted to the Board of Directors until it got final Board approval.

The team solved the problem by breaking down the factors that often made the Board have to go back and forth within the system. We looked into what was preventing an application from being turned in with everything clean and complete and then immediately being sent to the Board. Then we looked to decrease the cycle time from when the Board asked for more information until the Board representative received it. The team looked at how to decrease the number of incomplete applications and how to answer questions better (and faster) so that applications could be put before the Board more quickly.

PREVENTING TAMPERING

Without tools like Ishikawa diagrams, the system may lurch from pole to pole. We would introduce more variation, because every change made in response to a terrible case or an angry e-mail just confuses things and prevents reaching the root cause of the problem. As is often the case in medicine, the squeaky wheel definitely gets the grease. If you have a powerful person or group that squeaks often, a lot changes. It shouldn't, but that's typically what we do. We end up tampering with the system and almost always make the problem worse. Tampering with a system because we thought something was wrong (when it wasn't wrong) is a type 1 error.

When we use the Lean Six Sigma tools, we avoid constantly committing type 1 errors, where we think a difference exists when there isn't one. Type 1 errors, also known as alpha errors, are prevented by using statistical testing. When you make the choice to follow wherever the numbers take you, you avoid tampering with systems that may or may not need it. You avoid accidentally introducing more variation and making the quality much worse. The same goes for type 2 errors, where you think there's no difference when in fact there is one. Only good data can tell you if an issue is real and needs correction.

Once you have meaningful data, perform statistical testing to determine whether you're really seeing something different or whether it's just a fantasy. Your gut may be telling you you're doing better when you aren't (and thus missing opportunities). Statistical analysis will tell you if your gut is right. It will also keep you from charging uselessly at windmills with lance drawn as you misidentify items as issues that aren't.

You wouldn't change the variables in a chemistry experiment halfway through. The same is true when you do a quality-improvement study. If you start making changes ahead of the data, you change the experiment, and the results aren't valid. Of course, in medicine we don't like to think we're doing experiments on our patients—and patients don't like the idea of being experimented on. But when you apply Lean Six Sigma statistical testing techniques to quality improvement, you're not really experimenting in the sense of a medical trial. You're not experimenting on individual patients in any way. All you're doing is applying statistical process control to a system to make it work better. Once I learned about these tools, I began to believe that failure to use them is an alternative that's much worse. Blindly making changes has much more risk and so we never make any meaningful progress. In other words, learning about these tools but failing to use them seems much worse to me from the standpoint of risks to patients.

From the ethical standpoint, when I do a quality-improvement project I strongly encourage the group to include bounce-back—patients who return to the hospital quickly for the same problem or a related one—as an important measurement. We want to make sure bounce-back doesn't change as a result of whatever we're doing. If we do a project to shorten the time to discharge, for instance, we need to make very sure we're not getting more bounce-back.

That would indicate we're discharging people prematurely or that somehow our tweak to the system is having consequences we don't want.

Let's say a quality-improvement project has six parameters. You make changes, and five of the parameters improve and the sixth gets worse. You haven't achieved 100 percent success, but, depending on what they are, you can often see that the project worked. It's a victory. The endpoints you thought were the most desirable may not work out as well as you hoped, but any project will always be a mixed bag in that respect. It's not always as simple as "everything got better." Because healthcare is still in the dark ages on this stuff, however, typically everything does get better—because there were so many defects to begin with.

Part of the reason for this is simply that paying attention is really important. Attention alone gets you a certain amount of mileage. This is known as the Hawthorne effect or the observer effect: individuals change their behavior when they know they're being observed. The problem is, when you take away the project, the Hawthorne effect dissipates. You'll tend to see everything slip back to the way it was before. That's why the control phase of DMAIC is so important. The Hawthorne effect isn't necessarily a bad thing. We always say, "Well, look, if this is just the

Hawthorne effect and it's not a real improvement, we'll take it." I'll take the Hawthorne effect if it causes improvements, but I'm looking for sustainable improvement.

The Hawthorne effect was originally observed in the 1950s among factory workers. A hospital isn't exactly a factory. Among other things, it has a lot of built-in inefficiencies that no other business would ever tolerate (at least not a successful business). That's in part why there can be a lot of turmoil when business-minded people take over hospitals.

Reputation is one thing; results are another. This book exists, in part, because medical centers are highly resistant to looking objectively at ourselves with standard quality tools. We'll say things like, "Healthcare is not manufacturing," as if the tools we discuss here are specific to (and only work in) manufacturing—which, of course, isn't the case. The tools here don't care which process you use them on. They function well once they are applied properly.

I'm not sharing this to slam my colleagues or our industry, of which I'm very proud. We help a lot of people. With that said, we have been lagging behind other industries in how we handle quality; and thus this new value focus is making waves. Lean Six Sigma systems have been rare (I've previously been pretty lonely in quality meetings), but starting in 2014, those systems have become *much* more common in the industry.

Getting people to see and accept how they're really performing as a team, as opposed to how they think or wish they're performing, is a very tough conversation. In some cultures, healthcare staff may be afraid to take a square look at performance and make changes. We may worry about losing our reputation and our job. This is especially so because we very commonly have never heard of these tools and have no idea how to use them. Worse yet, when we do learn about data, we are often focused on the weaknesses we may see in our professional literature, rather than on how to use good data to make meaningful changes. The purpose of this book is to give us the vocabulary to have conversations about quality using standard tools in a productive way that gets results. It's doable, I promise. I've seen organizations improve by leaps and bounds in value delivery by adopting the mentality of data-driven improvement and using the expertise required to implement standard quality tools.

CHAPTER 6

DON'T JUST GET GOING—SIT THERE AND PLAN!

This time, the surgeon was late for his weekly coffee meeting with the hospital administrator. "Sorry," he said. "My turn to get hung up in a meeting that ran long. The data-collection part of a project is so important that I like to be sure everyone in the group gets it before we end the meeting."

"Tell me about it," said the administrator. "Sometimes I don't understand how a bunch of smart doctors can be so dense. This one doc in the pathology department keeps insisting we

need to study a problem that only comes up maybe once every couple of months. I see his point, because when it happens it's serious, but I don't know how to explain that there won't be enough data to make the results mean anything."

"You need to discuss sample size with the team," said the surgeon. "Get your Lean Six Sigma black belt to run through the sample-size equations with them. They're not that hard to grasp. Once they understand how to decide on the right sample size, they'll see immediately the right way to collect the data so that they do mean something. Set up your data collection the right way, and you improve the odds of success. Do it wrong, and your project will die a painful death."

✦ ✦ ✦

In the Department of Surgery, we're always trying to improve operating-room factors. Utilization time is a good example. Your OR may be up and running for elective cases from 7:00 or 7:30 a.m. until maybe 5:00 or 5:30 p.m. with full-time staffing, but you might only actually be operating on patients for 60 or 70 percent of the time. When you're not operating, the room is being turned over to be ready for the next patient. Turnover time isn't exactly value-added time, so you want to turn the room around as quickly but also as safely and completely as possible. It's necessary to do it correctly for safety, but it's not something for which a third-party payer will pay directly. Also, the time your OR sits empty (but is staffed to run) is nonvalue-added time, because it's work for which no third-party payer will pay your hospital. You also want to have the first cases of the day start on time.

So, if you want to do a study to figure out a more efficient way to schedule your OR usage, the first thing to decide (after you build the team for the project) is exactly what you're going to measure and define it accurately—part of the D in the DMAIC acronym. In this case, you would need to define turnaround time—when does it start and when does it end? When one patient is wheeled out and the next wheeled in? Or when the crew begins and ends the turnover work? What does start on time mean? When the patient is first brought in to the OR? Or when the surgeon arrives?

The next crucial step is create a data-collection plan, which includes deciding how big a sample you need. If you don't do these two things as some of your first steps, you have *no* shot at knowing how much data you have to collect to show a meaningful improvement or how long the improvement is going to take. With an insufficient sample size, you can end up with a project that will never have an answer or will be misleading. Unfortunately, most quality-improvement projects in healthcare don't consider sample size and so fumble at the kickoff. In part that's because a lot of projects seem to be done more to make people feel good or to show motion (look busy) than to come up with a statistically significant, meaningful improvement. Or perhaps it's just that staff don't know what it takes to demonstrate meaningful improvement. Those are direct, tough comments, I know, but they're true. Value improvements are arguably more important in healthcare than other fields. We're talking about taking care of people here. Aren't we obligated to deliver real, sustainable improvements in the value we deliver to patients, rather than performing projects that don't work?

HOW MUCH DATA IS ENOUGH?

To see whether you're really doing better, to know if you should celebrate success or wail over failure, you have to know how much data you need. The way you decide on a sample-size calculation in your data-collection plan is pretty easy. When you do a sample-size calculation, as we'll see in the next chapter, ask yourself, "What is the smallest change I want to be able to detect?" If you decide you want to be able to detect a 10 percent change, then you need less data than if you want to detect a 5 percent change as your smallest detectable, meaningful change. At the start, set how granular you want your detection scheme to be.

Once you've determined the smallest minimal change you want to be able to detect, you can calculate your sample size. If you have historic data from earlier studies, you can extrapolate from that. You might know from previous studies, for example, that you'll need about 60 patients to be able to draw meaningful conclusions. If you have a substantial sample size, this guards against premature celebration of success or lamentation of failure. It tells you to be patient before you make a lot of changes to a system all at once. It tells you to gather enough data to say meaningfully whether you're doing better or not. (The equations for how to decide your sample size aren't that complex. Your Lean Six Sigma black belt can help you work them out or do them for you. I'll go into the details in chapter 7.)

WHO COLLECTS THE DATA?

Your quality-improvement team has come up with a good project. Now someone needs to collect the data. That's actually something of a problem in most healthcare organizations. We don't usually have robust data-collection ability or the sophistication to interpret the data we do collect. That's why you probably need to bring in an expert Lean Six Sigma black belt. The black belt is trained to guide you through a data-collection plan.

The first question for the team is to decide what is the smallest change you want to see. If a 5 or 10 percent change would be meaningful, the team has set the parameters for what success looks like. A good data-collection plan will provide enough information to see if the desired change has been achieved.

If you don't set up a good data-collection plan, you're doomed.

The sophistication to interpret the data is key; so are the people around the process. Eighty percent of Lean Six Sigma is people. Only 20 percent is math, but that 20 percent is essential. How you set the stage to collect that 20 percent is key. Start with a very clear operational definition of the metric you're looking at. If it's time, for instance, when does the clock start and stop? What directionality do you want this metric to have? Is it better if the metric decreases ("smaller is better") or increases ("larger is better")?

It's possible that the importance of setting things up properly can be overstated—but very unlikely. The key to meaningful results is a good sample of appropriate size that collects data on the entire process. That means data from the times when it may be tougher to collect, such as nights and weekends. Getting the data may mean that you personally have to stand there with a stopwatch. If that's what it takes, then that's what you have to do.

Whenever possible, I suggest you avoid using data from trauma registries and data warehouses. The information you get has almost always been scrubbed in some way—it's probably been cleaned, edited, or otherwise filtered. Whenever possible, we recommend getting data directly from the process. In Lean Six Sigma terms, that means going to the *gemba*—the place where the process happens—to get a real feel for how it works. Assign someone to observe, talk to the participants, get a sense of what goes on, and then sit down and actually collect the data.

Knowing the limits of your data is important. Were the samples representative of the system at which you're looking? Is the sample size adequate to detect the size of the change for which you're looking?

USING THE SIPOC DIAGRAM

Remember the SIPOC diagram I discussed back in chapter 4? Let's put it to use again. We can use the suppliers, input, process, output, and customers information in the diagram to create the data-collection plan. In general, to fully characterize your system you will require six or seven endpoints. That's all. You don't need twenty data points—just six or seven are plenty for most quality-improvement projects. The diagram helps you narrow down your process-input endpoints to just one or two, your process endpoint to just one, and your process-output endpoints to just two or three. These endpoints are key to describe your system adequately.

Look at the SIPOC diagram with your group to see each element of the process. Choose the endpoints the group agrees have meaning for that element. In healthcare, we often run into an issue here. It's hard to believe, given how much data we see and track all the time, that we need so few endpoints to make dramatic improvement. *Believe it*. We don't need to be data rich and information poor for our quality-improvement projects, even though we may be used to that in the rest of our work. As a team leader, I've found it's always a challenge to focus the group on narrowing our view to the six or seven required endpoints. The reward for choosing a small number of endpoints is that the project tends to succeed.

Sometimes we can "double dip" the data. One endpoint can actually do double duty and represent two elements of your system. For example, sometimes we need to use trauma registry data or other data that has already been collected just because it's very handy, easy to get, and does what we need. Sometimes an element from a registry can serve as both an input measure and a process measure. Although I recommend avoiding registry data whenever possible, there are times when we can use it and even double dip with it. On rare occasions, you can use data from earlier projects in the same center.

DISCRETE AND CONTINUOUS DATA

How much data you need will depend on whether you decide to go with discrete or continuous data. I'll go into the distinctions in the next chapter. For now, let's just say continuous data is probably the best approach for most quality-improvement studies, because you can do a lot more with a lot less data when it's continuous instead of discrete. Your Lean Six Sigma black belt can apply the right equations to help you determine how much data you will need to characterize your system in order to detect a certain size change. At this point, in other words, the black belt can help you calculate what sample size you will need, based in part on the smallest meaningful change you would like to be able to detect. You absolutely must figure these things out before you collect data. Bear in mind that trying to detect a smaller change means you need many more data points.

DATA FIRST

Without Lean Six Sigma tools, the healthcare world looks very much as it does now: we have a lot of undulations in quality. We think we're doing better, but we're not sure. I sit through a lot of meetings where we look at problems, look at quality-improvement projects, look at results, and still don't know if whatever we tried to improve really is better. Sometimes you realize you're not measuring things that matter. That happens. The old saying is right on: "Without data, you just have an opinion."

The lesson is to gather data first. The data-collection plan is the central feature of good, quality projects. Before you start collecting the data, get everybody aligned on the same page for what "good" looks like. Get everybody aligned on what "improvement" looks like.

One problem with the data in any quality-improvement project is that you usually can't compare it to other projects. The endpoints that matter are changeable. Unless you adopt an operational definition that's exactly the same as the study you're looking at, you usually can't translate what you've done with these projects and the improvement you've made based on it into other hospital centers. You learn pretty quickly that the vagaries of what some other center did aren't always applicable to what your center does. You discover that what's called an apple in another hospital's study usually isn't what you call an apple, and vice versa. So, before you benchmark against other centers, I recommend you learn how to shine up the apples on your own apple cart first.

You can take ideas from other centers, but at your hospital it becomes about doing better with what you have. Once you've improved everything as much as possible, then you can benchmark against other centers. Magically, once your center is on the path toward continuously improving its own apples, that center begins to perform very well on external benchmarks.

WHAT ARE THE RIGHT ENDPOINTS?

When we look at something like turnaround times in the OR, we want to compare them to an industry standard. For example, for OR utilization time, 85 percent is pretty typical. The goal of your quality-improvement project might be to do better than that. But over time you find out it's not about where you start; it's about where you end up. You want to see improvement over time. Again, you also have to make sure that your study is talking about the same thing as the benchmark studies if you want to compare apples when you're done. Interestingly, even something as intuitively straightforward as OR utilization time may not be defined in the same way among the various studies, and it may not be defined in the same way you've chosen. Some centers, for example, may not consider turnaround time. They may define OR time not from the time the patient exits the room but from the time the nurse puts in the order that transfers the patient to the recovery unit. Definitions can be surprisingly ambiguous!

Some projects lend themselves better to Lean Six Sigma analysis than others. What we want to do are projects that are worth the time and effort. You're asking important people to take time from whatever else they're doing and to meet with you on an ongoing basis for months—the median time to get one of these projects done in health-care is three to four months, or often about 120 days. The productivity you're losing by asking them to do the project has to be justified by the return. It often is, because (again) median return on a quality-improvement project is usually about $250,000 in waste recovered over a single year. Before proposing any new quality-improvement project, I ask myself, "Is this worth $250,000?"

Let's say you improve the turnaround time in your ORs by 15 percent. Does that work out to be $250,000? It's sometimes hard to tell, because every organization values a minute of OR time differently. Some organizations say that to keep the OR doors open costs eighty dollars a minute. Others say it costs fifty-seven dollars a minute.

Those numbers are useful for giving you an estimate of the cost of poor quality and can help you decrease waste, improve turnaround times, stock the right supplies, and so on. In general, for expensive areas such as the OR, quality-improvement projects do pay off, because small savings in cost and efficiency add up proportionately faster. It's often surprisingly easy to achieve those savings.

CHAPTER 7

CONTINUOUS VS. DISCRETE DATA

At their usual weekly meeting for coffee in the little second-floor café, the hospital administrator and the surgeon were both feeling tired out by their quality-improvement efforts. They had been working hard to convince everyone that going from volume to value was the way forward for better quality. They had already shown the way with some successful projects that had really visible results. In fact, they had done such a good job that every department in the hospital was now clamoring for a Lean Six Sigma black belt to help them with their project ideas.

"One good project, and suddenly everybody has an idea. I've got a ton of quality proposals piling up on my desk," grumbled the hospital administrator. "Some of them are well thought out, but it's a little disappointing to see how many want to do the data collection in the wrong way. I'm pretty sure that if we did the project their way, we'd get the wrong answers. Isn't there some Lean Six Sigma terminology for that?"

"Do you mean type 1 and type 2 errors?" the surgeon asked.

"Yes, that's it. Thanks for jogging my memory. Now let me see if I can remember what they are. Type 1 errors mean you think you made a difference but you didn't, and type 2 errors mean you think there's no difference but there really is. Am I close?"

"You got it. How you collect the data makes all the difference in avoiding both kinds of errors."

✦ ✦ ✦

At one hospital I helped, a quality-improvement team wanted to see if they could improve the treatment of patients who needed to go directly to the operating room from the emergency department as quickly as possible. The goal was to improve the percentage of these patients who got to the OR in less than two hours. In a study such as this, you need to figure out what your endpoint will be.

The team chose to use a percentage of the total number of these emergency patients—what's called a discrete data endpoint. They opted for a percentage outcome because they wanted to show a meaningful, statistically significant improvement with a percentage they were used to seeing. (That hospital loved dashboards with percentages.) They wanted to know if they were doing better, and they felt that by using something like a percentage, which was very familiar to them, they could see if no change was happening. They wanted to avoid committing a type 1 error, thinking a difference exists when it doesn't, and a type 2 error, thinking there's no difference when in fact there is.

A problem immediately arose. Over the course of a year, there just weren't that many emergency patients who need to go right to the OR. The team was studying something that happened at most forty-five times (at that small center) a year. Because they had such a small number, their study was underpowered—they weren't able to show significant improvement. When they set up the data-collection plan, they set it up in such a way that they could never reach statistical significance. Why? Because they chose a discrete endpoint. Take this point home: Discrete data endpoints (such as percentages) usually take *many* more events/samples than non-discrete or continuous endpoints to allow you to tell whether there has been a significant improvement.

CATEGORIZING DATA

We can categorize data in a lot of ways, but two of the most useful are discrete and continuous. Discrete data is yes/no, black/white, stop/go, ABC—data that comes in little packets. Continuous data is data you can infinitely divide and have it still make sense. You can divide an hour into 60 minutes. You can divide a minute into 60 seconds. You can divide seconds into nanoseconds. Continuous data is usually preferable to discrete data for quality-improvement projects, because you can do a lot more with a lot less of it.

Let's think about that failed OR study. What if the study had simply tracked time to the OR for these patients? By simply tracking time, you could say whether you had or had not made a statistically significant improvement. The study still might not have enough patients for a discrete data endpoint, but you're more likely to get useful information by seeing if you can minimize the time rather than reduce the percentage that took longer than some amount of time.

How you ask the question is really key. By using discrete data to track the patients, the quality team ended up making the mistakes they wanted to avoid. In my experience, when discrete data is used where continuous data would be more helpful, you end up in meeting after meeting talking about what you have to do differently for a process. Worse yet, someone may say in the meeting that the process is fine, when in fact it's not. You make both errors because you're using the wrong question with the wrong data.

ASK THE RIGHT QUESTION

One important point of this book is to make sure you start asking the right questions. Setting up the question properly allows us to really know if we are doing better delivering quality and value to our patients.

If you can, involve professionals, such as Lean Six Sigma black belts, right from the start. Black belts are trained in data collection and analysis and in statistical process control. In fact, that's what statistical process control is designed to do: to guard against the thought errors we commonly make. Your black belt can keep you on the right track to ask the right questions. If you use statistical safeguards, it's possible that you'll walk forward more slowly, but it's less likely you'll end up walking backward on your quality journey without knowing you're doing it!

Setting up the data-collection plan, as I discussed in the last chapter, and calculating how many patients or items (or whatever you're studying) you'll need is much more powerful and useful than almost any other step in the process. It tells you exactly what you need to know to achieve success with your project. It tells you how long the project is going to take, how many people need to be in it, how much of what sort of data you need to collect, and more. Work with a Lean Six Sigma black belt if you can; if not, this chapter will help you figure out how to do the data collection correctly on your own.

If you set your project up correctly to begin with, it's likely to run smoothly and give you actionable results. I always remind myself of the old adage "Spend time now, save time later." If you set up the data-collection phase of the project wrong, it's difficult to recover. One reason is that you won't know you've created a problem for yourself until you start doing the statistical testing once all the data has been collected. You'll see only then that you either haven't made any progress or you have made progress. If you haven't made any progress because you don't have a sample that ever allows you to show progress, it's really hard to figure that out, because from what you see you will think, "Oh, I didn't make any progress." It's no surprise you didn't make any progress—you don't have an adequate sample, or you chose a discrete data endpoint that requires an inordinate amount of time that you'll never be able to reach or your project just doesn't have.

In health-care quality projects, these questions aren't usually even on the radar. That's a huge problem, because doing a project without using these safeguards can actually be dangerous. You start correcting problems that don't exist, but you're not correcting or even seeing problems that sometimes do exist. Intuition can really mislead us. The errors in a project that's set up incorrectly might only be detected months later, when everybody is really frustrated. Sometimes the result of a project is "Well, we just weren't successful," which can happen even when the project is set up correctly. But what can also happen is that the project did make a difference but you just can't detect it or prove it.

WHY CONTINUOUS DATA IS BETTER

In quality-improvement projects, continuous data is almost always going to be better than discrete data. One more time (I'm sure you're singing along by now): the reason is that continuous data need a much smaller sample to show meaningful change. We can show this by looking at the sample-size equations for both types of data.

Here's the equation for how big a sample of discrete data is needed to allow meaningful detection of a certain size change. Notice that you specify what that "smallest detectable change" is when you set up the project and the sample size. In other words, you get to make choices that impact how large a sample you will need.

$$(p)\ (1 - p)\ (2/delta)^2$$

This sample-size equation for discrete data has several important consequences. First, consider the terms. *P* is the probability of outcome of a certain event. This is for percentage-type data where we have a yes/no or stop/go or similar data point, so *p* is the probability of the event occurring. The *delta* is the smallest change we want to be able to detect with our sample.

The 2 in the equation comes from the (approximate) z-score at the 95 percent level of confidence. (The z-score is also called the standard score. It indicates how many standard deviations an element is from the mean.) We round up from the true value of *z* to 2 because that gives us a whole-number sample slightly larger than what's required, rather than a sample with a fraction in it or one that's a bit too small. (How can you have 29.2 patients, for example?) Rounding up is important, because rounding down would yield a sample that may be slightly too small.

Let's say we have an event that has a 5 percent probability of occurring. This would be fairly typical for many things in medicine, such as wound infections under certain circumstances. When we work through the equation to figure out the sample size we need to detect a 2 percent change in that percentage, we have 0.05 × 0.95 (2/0.02)². This gives us approximately 475 samples required in order to detect the smallest possible decrease of 2 percent. In other words, we have to get a fairly large sample size to see a reasonable change. We can't detect a change of just 1 percent with that sample size. So, if we think we see 4.8 percent as the new percentage after interventions to reduce the number of wound infections, then because of our sample size, we probably can't really say if anything has changed in terms of that percentage.

Now let's look at the same quality-improvement goal using continuous data. The sample size required to detect some delta at 95 percent level of confidence can be represented as follows:

([2][historic standard deviation of the data]/delta)²

Remember, as with the discrete data equation, you set the delta as the smallest change you want to be able to find. When we plug the numbers into this simplified sample-size equation, we see very quickly that we come out with much smaller samples of data required to show significant change.

SOME HANDY TIPS

If you don't know the probability of an event because you've never measured it before, just make your best guess. A good starting point if you have no idea, and have reason to believe that what you're looking at is just as likely to happen as it is *not* to happen, is to consider 0.5 as the p. Some sample-size calculation is better than none in many ways. You can always revise the p as you start to collect data from the system and you get a sense of what the p actually is.

If you don't know the historic standard deviation of your data (or you don't have one), take the highest value of your continuous data and subtract the lowest. Divide what you get by 3. This rule of thumb gives you a quick estimate of historic standard deviation. As you collect more data over more projects, you can replace the estimate with more accurate information. If you have an estimate of your historic standard deviation based on data from previous studies, you can use that.

Ordinarily, you would have a standard deviation in your continuous data equation. Not all data sets have a standard deviation, however, because not all data sets are normal. Some aren't normally distributed. The details of that are beyond the scope of this book, but what you need to know is that nonnormal data can be changed to fit the normal curve and give you a standard deviation. The mathematical process doesn't fudge the data; it changes it, just as water can be changed to ice. It's still water, just in a different physical form.

PUTTING THE EQUATIONS TO USE

Let's say we want to track whether a patient is seen by an ED doctor within thirty minutes of checking in with the triage nurse. We start out already knowing that the probability of this is 50 percent and stating that we want to have the ability to detect a 10 percent improvement. We really set the project up to be only as granular as being able to detect a large change such as 10 percent—anything smaller, and we'd probably miss it. How big does your sample size need to be in order to have a smallest detectable change of something (large) like 10 percent?

Using the discrete sample equation (p) (1 – p) (2/delta)^2, the numbers would be 0.50 (1 – 0.50) (2/0.10)^2. Work it out to detect a 10 percent change, and you find you want an estimated sample size of about 100.

Let's pretend the smallest change you'd be willing to accept is 5 percent, not 10 percent. If you plug the numbers in, you see that you're going to need a much bigger sample to detect that smaller change.

What if you didn't have the time to get through a one-hundred-patient sample? In that case, you could use continuous data and get real results from fewer patients, because you would need fewer data points. If you plug the numbers into the continuous sample equation ([2] [historic standard deviation of the data]/delta)^2, you'll see the difference.

Let's say the standard deviation is five minutes, and we want to be able to detect any change in the system as small as two minutes. That's a sample of twenty-five patients. Of course, we want to be sure whatever sample we take represents the full system—not just one great shift that an ER physician had on a Tuesday during the daylight hours! Remember to represent nights and weekends in your sample.

Notice that using continuous data often lets you end the project sooner. Discrete data can make a project really drag on because it can take longer to gather the endpoints. You could be collecting discrete data for a long time before you have any idea of what's going on.

UNLOCKING TOOLS WITH CONTINUOUS DATA

Another reason continuous data is preferable to discrete data is the number of powerful tools it unlocks. Continuous data allows us to use many other quality tools, such as data power transforms and useful hypothesis testing, that are more challenging with discrete data. Your Lean Six Sigma black belt can help you understand and use these statistical tools to get more distance out of your data.

Having a continuous data endpoint also lets you create better visual representations. It allows the team to visualize the robustness of the process along with the current level of variation in the process. Visual representation can be more challenging with discrete data endpoints.

A CAUTIONARY TALE

Once upon a time there was a department of surgery that wanted to improve its use of a surgical safety checklist. The quality-improvement team believed this would help keep patients safer in their surgical system. The team decided to use discrete data to assess whether the checklist was being used appropriately. When they drew up their data-collection plan, they decided a checklist missing any element at all (and there were *lots* of elements) would be called "not adequate." If it was 100 percent complete in all elements, it would count as "adequate." The team's target goal was to have 100 percent of checklists considered adequate.

The team collected data on the department of surgery's current performance and found that only 40 percent of checklists were adequate. Clearly, something needed to be done to improve compliance. The team made some changes to the checklist that they thought would help, such as requiring the surgeon to be present on the patient's physical arrival in the operating room.

They were very eager to see how well the changes would work. They had posed the question as a binary one: the checklist would be either 100 percent complete (adequate) or less than 100 percent complete (inadequate). They wanted to detect significant changes of at least 10 percent or larger in the system. To determine how large their sample size needed to be, they used the discrete data formula. The formula estimated a sample size of ninety-six.

Weeks later, when they had finally reached ninety-six samples, the team reviewed the data to discover how much things had improved. Experientially, the team saw that many more checklists were used and that there was significantly more participation. It had taken a while to get to ninety-six samples, and the team was ready to celebrate. Much more of the checklist was being completed each time. But when the team used their numbers in statistical testing, the numbers showed no significant improvement in checklist utilization. Why was that?

They asked the question in the wrong way. And because they framed the question in the wrong way, they had used a discrete data endpoint, which required a large sample and made it difficult to demonstrate the improvement that the team really believed they had made. Here's what happened.

Anything other than complete checklist utilization went into the "not adequate" bin and was counted against them. So, even if the checklists were much more complete than they ever had been (and that seemed to be so), anything less than perfection still counted against the percentage of complete (adequate) checklists. Because they used discrete data in that way, they were unable to demonstrate significant improvement based on their numbers. It even seemed that more of the checklists were adequate (100 percent complete) than ever before, yet maybe it was only 5 percent more than previously. Where prior to changes most checklists were missing five to ten elements, now they were only missing one or two. It seemed as if improvements had been made, but because of the way the question and sample were framed, it was difficult to demonstrate. The team was disappointed that the project had "failed," even though they had actually made great strides in improving checklist utilization.

If the team had designed a continuous data endpoint for

checklist completion, they would have required a smaller sample size that could have shown meaningful improvement more easily and sooner. Maybe they could have intervened to get checklists completely filled out (made "adequate"), instead of waiting to reach the sample size of ninety-six checklists.

As the story shows, discrete data endpoints can limit your ability to demonstrate meaningful change in several important ways. In addition to misleading us when we don't know enough to use statistical testing, discrete data may also delay improvements as we wait to build a sample. Continuous data, by contrast, can allow teams such as the checklist team to demonstrate significant improvement even if checklists are still not quite 100 percent complete. Your choice of endpoints can greatly impact your ability to draw meaningful conclusions as well as your chance of celebrating meaningful change. As we move from volume to value, it's important to have the expertise to know not only *what* to measure but *how* to measure it.

CHAPTER 8

STOP LYING TO YOURSELF AND GET TO THE REAL ROOT CAUSE

At their weekly coffee meeting in the little second-floor café, the hospital administrator asked the surgeon to move to a more secluded table in a back corner. After they settled in, the administrator said, "I asked to move back here so we won't be overheard. I wanted to talk to you about dealing with personnel."

The surgeon said, "Good idea to keep it quiet, although nothing stays quiet in a hospital for long. What's your concern?"

The administrator responded, "You know, now that I've been looking at quality issues in the hospital for a while, I can see that there's a lot of variability. I guess that's to be expected in something so people-centered as healthcare, but really, isn't there a way to cut back on it? The department heads I talk to say this program or that is going well, but then staff members buttonhole me in the corridors to complain about the same program. The department heads tell me the program is fine and doesn't need to be looked at, but they can't tell me why they think that's so. I really need a way to get them to rethink the need for data."

"They're not lying to themselves when they say a program is chugging along well, but they're not being completely honest with themselves either. That's always a problem," the surgeon said. "We all like to think we're doing a good job. We also don't like having to scrutinize our programs, because it's hard to stay objective when we do. Often, people start feeling threatened or blamed even when we're very careful to leave individuals out."

"I can see that happening every time I bring this stuff up," the administrator replied. "Everyone gets very defensive, as if I'm going to fire them on the spot."

The surgeon said, "I've found that doing a root-cause analysis, where you look as directly as you can at all the variables, such as whether the computers are running slowly too often or if there's a lot of staff turnover in the ICU, can really help people see problems objectively, not personally. It really lays the problems out and lets you see where the changes should be."

+ + +

I was recently part of a team that was trying to decide how well residents in our hospital were supervised. The issue is important, because residency programs are required to have excellent oversight to maintain their certification. Senior physicians are supposed to supervise the residents as the residents care for patients. There are also supposed to be regular meetings with the residents and meaningful oversight during patient care. We had to be able to show accrediting agencies that supervision was happening effectively. Everyone on the team, myself included, felt we really did well with residents in terms of supervision. We would answer their questions, help them out with patients in the middle of the night, and do everything we could to guide them in providing safe, excellent patient care. At least, we thought we did.

We would have meetings and say, "The resident was supervised because we did this with him and we had that conversation about a patient." None of this was captured anywhere; it was all subjective feelings on the part of the senior medical staff. The residents, however, were telling us that they felt supervision could have been better in the overnight shifts and also in some other specific situations. Still, we (especially the senior staff doing the supervising) would tell ourselves in the meetings, "We're doing a good job. We know we're supervising them well."

We weren't lying to ourselves. We were supervising the residents pretty well. We just couldn't demonstrate it in the ways that mattered, and we were concerned about any perceived lack in the overnight supervision. We were having plenty of medical decision-making conversations with the residents and helping them in all the ways we were supposed to, but we didn't have a critical way to evaluate our efforts in terms of demonstrating how we were doing or having something tangible to improve.

When I say, "Stop lying to yourself," I refer to how we tend to self-delude ourselves into thinking that things are OK, even when they're not. How would we ever know? What changes our ability to think about our performance? Data. When good data tell us, objectively and without question, that something has to change, we have to agree. Having good data prevents all of us from thinking we're above average—a common misconception.

To improve our resident supervision, we first had to agree that it needed improvement. To reach that point, we had to collect data prospectively and review it. But before we even thought about data collection, we had to deal with the unspoken issue of protection. We had to make sure all the attending physicians knew they were protected against being blamed, scapegoated, or even fired if the data turned out to show problems. We had to reassure everyone that we weren't looking for someone to blame. We were looking for ways to make a good system better. There are ways to collect data that are anonymous. The way we chose did not include which attending physician or resident was involved at each data point. That protection was key (and is *very* important in quality-improvement projects in healthcare) to allowing the project to move ahead.

I've found it helps to bring the group to the understanding that it is wrong to think that, because we are so good, data collection on the process will show us that we're just fine—maybe even that we are exceptionally good. Usually, once the data are in, that's not the case. On the rare occasion when the system really is awesome, I help the group to go out of its way to celebrate and to focus on what can be replicated in other areas to get that same level of success.

When we collected the data on resident supervision, we asked ourselves the Five Whys (check back to chapter 5 for more on this). Why do we think we may not be supervising residents well? What tells us that? The documentation is not very good. Why is the documentation not very good? We can't tell if it doesn't reflect what we're doing or if we don't have some way to get what we're doing on the chart. Why don't we have some way to get it on the chart? Well, because...

If you ask yourself the question "Why?" five times, chances are you'll get to the root cause of why things are the way they are. It's a tough series of questions. It requires self-examination. You have to be very honest and direct with yourself and your colleagues. You also have to know some of the different ways that things can be—you have to apply your experience and get ideas from others to see what is *not* going on in your system. Some sacred cows may lose their lives in the process. At other times you may run up against something missing from a system, an absence rather than presence of something like a sacred cow. What protections are *not* there? As the saying goes, "If your eyes haven't seen it, then your mind can't know it."

As we asked ourselves the Five Whys, we asked why we felt we were doing a good job but an outsider wouldn't be able to tell. We decided that the only way an outsider could ever know that we were supervising well was by making sure that supervision was thoroughly documented in the patient charts.

The next step was to collect data on our documentation to see how good it was. We decided to rate it on a scale of one to five. One was terrible: there is no sign of any documentation of decision-making or senior physician support in the chart. Five was great: we can really see that what we said was happening has happened.

We focused on why the decision-making process wasn't getting documented in the charts. There were lots of reasons: Because it's midnight. Because we're not near a computer. Because we were called away to another patient. Because the computers were down. Because the decision was complicated, and it was difficult to record it accurately.

We developed a system for scoring the charts that I felt was pretty objective. The data were gathered prospectively; names were scrubbed, because we didn't care which surgeon it was and we didn't want to bias the scoring. To validate the scoring, we used a Gage Reproducibility and Reliability test, which (among other things) helps determine how much variability in the measurement system is caused by differences between operators. We chose thirty charts at random and had three doctors check them and give them a grade with the new system. Each doctor was blinded to the chart they rated (as much as you could be) and rated each chart three times. We found that most charts were graded at 2 or 2.5.

Once we were satisfied that the scoring system was valid, we applied it prospectively and scored a sample of charts according to the sample-size calculation we had performed. Reading the chart to see if it documented supervision correctly only took about a second. We found, again, that our score was about 2.5. That was a little dismaying, because it showed we weren't doing as well as we thought, although we weren't doing terribly, either.

Then we came up with interventions that we thought would improve the score. We made poka-yoke changes—changes that made it easier to do the right thing without having to think about it. In this case, the poka-yoke answer was to make it easier to document resident oversight and demonstrate compliance with Physicians at Teaching Hospitals (PATH) rules; the changes made it harder to avoid documenting actions. By making success easier, we saw the scores rise to 5 and stay there. We added standard language and made it easy to access in the electronic medical record. We educated the staff. We demonstrated how, and why, it was easier to do the right thing and use the tool instead of skipping the documentation and getting all the work that resulted when the documentation was not present.

ROOT-CAUSE ANALYSIS

The project succeeded extremely well because we stopped lying to ourselves. We used data and the Five Whys to see that what we told ourselves didn't align with what was happening. We didn't start with the assumption that we were lying to ourselves. We thought we were doing a good job. We talked about what a good job looked like, how we'd know if we were doing a good job, and so on, but what really helped us put data on the questions was using a fishbone diagram. We used the diagram to find the six different factors of special cause variation. (Check back to chapter 5 for more on fishbone diagrams.)

We looked at all the five Ms and one P—the different factors that go into good resident supervision and that can cause variation in quality. The factors we brought out in this case were as follows:

- **People:** the individuals involved, how they interacted, and how they documented

- **Material:** the physical chart (could you even *find* that chart to write in it?) and how sick the patient was. After all, sometimes when we were with a very sick patient, we were appropriately focused on that patient and *not* as much on documenting resident supervision.

- **Machine:** computer availability for documentation

- **Method:** the documentation and supervision process

- **Mother Nature:** the impact of what's going on in the world, such as weather factors that increase the number of patients, our workload, and our ability to document well

- **Management:** who reads the charts to say whether we were doing a good job, and how well they look to find evidence of our supervision

Those data points go on the spines of the fishbone diagram. When you see them laid out in this way, they help you realize that the data is nothing personal. The solution isn't just "The doctor should work harder" or "The doctor needs to do more," which is our fallback for a lot in medicine. The fishbone diagram tells us that the system isn't set up for optimal results. It fact, it conspires toward an outcome that's not as good as it could be. The fishbone diagram reminds us that multiple holes in the Swiss cheese have to line up for something to happen, good or bad. If we cared enough to highlight an issue with resident supervision, isn't it worth using the tools to represent *everything* that went into making it what it was? Representing *all* the factors let us improve it. If you have a sacred cow you can't mention, it *will* get in the way.

When process-improvement programs aren't robust, culture is a huge driver. Everybody will tend to dance around the real problem, afraid they will get fired for bringing it up or get blamed (and fired) for causing it. As the great management thinker W. Edwards Deming said, "A bad system will beat a good person every time." There's another old saying that also applies here: "Culture eats strategy for breakfast." I'm not saying that quality-improvement efforts *must* be impolitic or confrontational. I'm just saying that the ability to discuss, collegially, difficult topics is a hallmark of a high-functioning quality-improvement program that helps deliver value to patients.

If the culture of the system is such that people are going to get into trouble of some sort by raising quality issues, your process-improvement system will be subverted. It will have no wind in its sails. That's why it's so important to make the process *only* about quality improvement. The participants need to be reassured that the data will be anonymous and random and used only for the intended purpose, not as an attack weapon. Nothing will be personally assignable, which is where a lot of quality projects in medicine break down. "Quality as a weapon" *must* be off the table.

Another concern that needs to be addressed is medical malpractice. The participants need to know that the process-improvement system is protected by peer review. In other words, the data are *anonymized and inaccessible.* They're protected (rules vary from state to state) and can't be subpoenaed for cases of medical malpractice and related issues. That's unfortunately not true or easy to achieve in every state, so this is something to check before beginning some types of projects. How will the data be protected? Are there any methods *beyond* the fact that they are anonymous?

GETTING TO THE ROOTS

A root-cause analysis (RCA) that uses a fishbone diagram takes people into account as one of the main elements. It shows that people are an important component, but also that the current system sets people up for certain outcomes. The real intent of the project isn't to blame anyone; it's simply to discover what aligned to make happen whatever happened. The intent is to learn from it and do better next time. The point of the exercise is to say, "OK, what opportunities do we have here? What system changes can we make? What personnel changes? What has to happen to do better next time?" It's not to focus on what an individual did wrong. We don't want to absolve someone who messes up from blame, but we also need to recognize that humans and human error are a component of the process-improvement system. And certain system issues (some of which we can modify and control) set us up for certain outcomes.

When we have a good root-cause analysis, the issues usually have multiple possible solutions. One of the least common is "Let's spend some money on it to fix the problem." Giving more resources to a bad system (as a lone solution) is rarely a potential answer that comes up from an RCA, but that's the solution that I do see chosen sometimes. When that is chosen as a lone intervention, I know the RCA probably didn't get to what really needs to happen for quality. Spending money and giving resources is a way to improve a system that's basically OK but could be better, yet it only gets us so far. Experientially speaking, I've found the most significant improvements come from thinking about how we do something differently rather than just spending "dumb money" on something.

Also, sometimes, other administrators involved have trouble seeing how giving resources translates into the bottom line. They don't see how the cost of poor quality means you recover much more when you really fix the problem and avoid defects than when you try to fix it with an inadequate budget and don't do well. Cheaping out isn't the way to solve a problem or improve a system either. In other words, allocating resources to something is one potentially important fix for a system, but by no means the only one. In modern healthcare, it's more important than ever to have a bigger tool set rather than simply to throw money at system problems.

The fishbone diagram is great for your root-cause analysis, but it's hard to see statistical significance, because it's often all intuitive, based on your gut feelings and experience. You think that these layers of the Swiss cheese lined up to create the defect, but which areas are really associated with this outcome? Could you tell which elements that the group came up with are *really* associated with this outcome? That's where the next level, multiple regression, comes in. If you do a multiple regression, it tells you which factors seem to correlate with the outcome so you know which ones to go after to really make a difference. This helps avoid a problem in healthcare, which is looking at things in isolation, being distracted by noise, and not focusing on system factors that actually had an impact.

With multiple regression, you use your data after the fact and ask, "Which of these factors actually correlates with this outcome?" Some of them will, and some of them won't. It tells you where to direct your energy.

When the fishbone diagram is combined with a multiple regression tool, the results can be very powerful. The math involved might seem daunting, but a Lean Six Sigma black belt or other consultant can handle it for you. Commercial software packages are available, but you'll get to the right answers sooner if you bring in an expert.

Multiple regression lets you segregate the factors and figure out what proportion of the variation you see is due to factors you can and can't control. The multiple regression helps reveal how much of variation is due to factors you can control. That helps you head in the right direction when you start making changes. And when variation is due to uncontrollable factors (noise), you want to know that, too. A good multiple-regression model shows that 80 percent of the variability in the outcome you're looking at is due to the factors you've included. These techniques can really show you which system factors provide value or are associated with high quality.

If you make the model and only 50 percent of the variability in outcome is due to the factors you included, that means you don't have all the right factors. You're missing something. Go back to the drawing board. There's something else at play you don't really understand or you haven't teased out. Once you have most of the factors associated with variability in your outcome, you can label which factors are controllable and which are noise.

If only 40 percent of the variability is due to controllable factors, but the overall model is 90 percent accurate, that means the model predicts very well what's going to go into this outcome. The model tells you that you've got the right factors, but only 40 percent of that variability is due to controllable factors. It doesn't mean you just throw your hands up in the air and stop. It just means you focus really hard on eliminating that 40 percent of the variability, because that's the best you'll ever be able to do under this model.

USING THE RESULTS

After all your work, the results come in and show that you had a good model. The next step is to meet with the team and ask, "Now, what do we do with this? What can we change? What are the controllable factors we can change? What do we need to change with those? What resources do we need, if any? What has to happen now?" To get these questions answered in an actionable way, make sure you've got all your stakeholders and decision-makers at the table.

I participated in a quality-improvement project that really showed me how applying multiple-regression analysis in combination with a fishbone diagram can have valuable application in the real world of healthcare.

Our trauma center had issues with excess time on "diversion," meaning that the ED was so full that we couldn't accept any additional patients. Of course, sometimes patients were still dropped off at our door or were very nearby to the hospital and so were brought in anyhow. We had to help those patients as best we could. As for other patients, we had to divert them to a different medical center. Over a fairly short time span, the center had more than two hundred hours of diversion—very undesirable in terms of quality of care and lost revenue.

The administration was floating multiple reasons for why so much diversion was needed. Possibilities included the idea that the ER physicians just weren't talented enough to avoid the situation. Other possible reasons included the weather (perhaps counterintuitively, if you've never worked in an ED, since EDs are busier on sunny days) or the lack of availability of regular hospital-floor beds.

The system was at a loss. Clearly, the first step was to get everyone on the same page about where to start and what to do next.

There's nothing like a fishbone diagram to clarify thinking. Some of the variables used in the diagram included the ER provider who was working when the diversion occurred, the day of the week, the weather, and the availability of ICU beds. The final regression result gave an r^2 value of less than 80 percent. However, the availability of ICU beds reached statistical significance. In other words, the model we had devised predicted less than 80 percent of the variability we saw in whether we were on diversion or not. As I described above, we really needed a better model. When we went back to the drawing board, we noticed that one item we had in our model *was* significantly associated with our time on diversion: availability of ICU beds.

We interpreted this to mean that the availability of ICU beds was significantly associated with whether the hospital was on diversion or not. Fewer ICU beds were associated with increased time on diversion. This gave us a tangible starting point to correct the issue. Why? Who knows exactly why? These models, in fact, don't answer why. They just tell us what the situation is. It's not causal thinking—it's statistical association. That fact can make it a bit uncomfortable at first if you're new to these tools.

Just as important was what the model *didn't* show. The diversion issue was *not* associated significantly with the ER doctors. Here's a good example of how data can help foster positive relationships. In this case, it took away the idea that the ER providers were somehow responsible for (or associated with) the diversion issue.

One obvious intervention was to expand the ICU in terms of available nursing staff. This allowed more staffed beds and made the ICU more available to accept patients. The diversion time issue led to an increased effort to recruit and retain critical-care nurses. The diversion challenge resolved immediately once the additional staff were available. Interestingly, the model as a whole didn't predict more than 80 percent of the variability seen in diversion, and yet once the one significant item (staffed ICU beds) was improved—poof!—the rest of the diversion issue disappeared.

CHAPTER 9

UNDERCONTROLLING: A TALE OF TWO ORGANIZATIONS

The surgeon was in a bad mood when the hospital administrator arrived for their weekly coffee meeting. "We had something go wrong in the OR today, and now the senior surgeon wants to shake up the entire restocking system. He gave me a hard time in front of the staff, and he's already fired off angry e-mails to just about everybody in the hospital."

"I know," said the administrator. "He even sent it to me. What should I do about it?"

"Just don't panic. When you rush into change because of one isolated event, you're likely to commit a type 1 error and fix what doesn't need fixing. Let's take his point seriously, but slow things down and look carefully at the system before we go tampering with it."

+ + +

The worst errors you can make in a quality-improvement program are type 1 and type 2 errors. A type 1 error finds a problem where none exists. A type 2 error fails to recognize a problem that does exist.

TYPE 1 ERRORS: IMAGINARY PROBLEMS

If I had to choose between an organization that makes type 1 errors and one that makes type 2 errors, I would choose the type 1 group. That organization may be tampering with its systems, finding problems where none exist, and overcorrecting small problems, but its heart is in the right place. Yes, it's often wasting its time, making work, and introducing more variability into a system (thus decreasing quality), but that organization *wants* to do better. It's got a chance to eventually figure out its issues and improve. Of the different organizations I've worked with, I like ones that do too much rather than too little. Every problem such organizations recognize may not be real, and they may overadjust, but at least they recognize they can improve.

I worked with one organization where there was such a strong desire to improve that they were all over the place with initiatives. They made horrible overreactions in response to just one bad case. They threw out entire processes and remade them without any thought about how that may actually introduce worse quality. They went through policy after policy because of outcomes that were suboptimal. We had tons of meetings that were really just wheel-spinning, without demonstrable increases in quality. It was a lot of work and actually brought us to worse outcomes.

RED LIGHT/GREEN LIGHT SYNDROME

In healthcare, we often measure things in percentages. When we track activities on a dashboard, we often change the colors to reflect changes in quality. Let's imagine a situation where we were trying to eliminate surgical wound infections in a small hospital. Imagine that, one month, 10 percent of our surgical patients developed wound infections. (This would probably never happen even in a bad hospital—I'm just using 10 percent to make the math easy.) On the dashboard for the medical staff, that number is shown in red because it's really bad. We want it to be very close to zero. Imagine that the next month the rate of wound infections is 0 percent. We're happy, and we turn the number green on the dashboard. The next month, the rate of wound infections shoots up to 10 percent again, and the dashboard turns red. Naturally, the staff is now asking, "What are we doing wrong? What happened? We've got to do something."

It turns out that there may be no significant statistical difference from month to month. If in one month no patient out of twenty has a surgical infection, then the infection rate is 0 percent. If the next month two patients out of twenty get an infection, then the monthly rate is suddenly 10 percent, but the number of patients with an infection is still small, especially when seen over a longer time frame. Over two months and forty patients, two patients with an infection means the rate is 5 percent—not great at all, but less horrifying than 10 percent.

The imaginary hospital may not be doing any worse when the dashboard goes from green to red or any better when it goes from red to green. It's possible that the hospital is perceiving differences that don't exist and overreacting to them by instituting new processes and then throwing them out again after talking for hours about how bad we are now or how good we are now. Knowing when to react and when not to react to avoid tampering is really tough.

The best way to recognize that you're tampering with a system that actually works pretty well is to use statistical testing with that discrete data. You have to make sure you have a big enough sample size to detect the change you're looking for. You've got to make sure the sample reflects everybody. It usually does, but at smaller hospitals, "everybody" over some time period may not be enough patients to determine if your system is any better (or worse) than it's ever been. Assuming your sample size is large and complete, you still need to do statistical testing, such as a chi-squared proportions test for percentage testing, to tell if you actually have a significant difference and if you should react or not.

When you tamper with a system, by definition you're making things worse. How can you tell when you've tampered instead of improved? That's where Lean Six Sigma really comes in. Assuming you've created a good data-collection plan, a range of statistical techniques can tell you if your data show anything has changed. Organizations that don't do this robustly or explicitly often have no idea if they're doing better. They just don't know. If we want to stop chasing our tails on quality-improvement projects, and to start meaningfully marching toward value over volume, we need to develop the sophistication to collect, process, and interpret our data.

I always like to know, when can I celebrate? When can I say that things are so much better than they were? I'm looking to celebrate successes, even small ones. I'm also looking to eliminate failure, and that comes out of statistical testing, too. You can see where you're not doing better and need to do more. That safeguard of testing is really useful for these situations.

Don't base your decision on data if you don't even have enough data. How do you know if you don't have enough? Again, you have to use the sample-size equation up front. You've got to do statistical testing on your pre- and post-state. That's how you protect yourself against tampering or missing a problem.

TYPE 2 ERRORS: UNRECOGNIZED PROBLEMS

Type 2 errors come from undercontrolling; it means there's a problem, but we missed it. These errors are tough to spot, because organizations often have a political climate or internal culture that can't recognize when it has issues. The organization may also lack the sophistication to use data correctly.

The way to avoid type 2 errors is to have a robust data-collection system and a robust process-improvement system. Both need to be staffed adequately with people who have the expertise to run studies and know what to do with data. Without that, you've got no shot at realizing that you're committing a type 2 error. You don't have any data to check yourself against. The power of data is that it can change your mind about what you think is going on, beyond your daily experience of a pathway.

In my experience, most organizations that undercontrol have "ostrich syndrome." Consciously or not, they put their head in the sand to ignore their problems. It's not usually the fault of one person. It's just that internal politics and culture conspire to keep the system from surfacing or correcting issues.

A common type 2 error happens when, for instance, the ED director comes to you every day and says, "We're overrun. We have patients who stay for hours. We've got to do something." Maybe you feel the organization doesn't have the money to do something about it, or doesn't have the resources in some other way. Or maybe you just don't believe the ED director because she's a good doctor but she's not a nice person and you think she complains a lot. The messenger effect makes you rule out what she's telling you; you dismiss her as just a complainer. This is easy to do because you also don't like her. Of course, maybe she's not a nice person to you because she's so exasperated by having this overcrowding problem go unacknowledged for so long. But because you don't like her and your budget is very tight, the issue doesn't even get surfaced.

Then one day an elderly sick lady waits in the ED for eight hours before getting treated. She eventually dies of sepsis in the hospital. Finally, the problem your ED director has been complaining about for months gets through to everyone in the administration, because the family sues. Because you didn't look into the problem and get data on it, you couldn't see it until something really bad happened and the lawyers got involved. The cost of poor quality is now very apparent: the hospital's reputation suffers, the staff morale suffers, the ED director is totally burned out and quits, regulators are asking questions, there's a big settlement, and the ED problem is now finally getting urgent—and therefore expensive—attention from outside consultants.

The death of a patient from languishing too long in the ED is a low-probability event with severe associated problems. Things that were supposed to happen for that patient didn't. In the full house of variation, almost every eventuality will manifest at some point on a long enough timeline. The question is, how can you make that timeline so long that a really bad event happens only very rarely?

Step one is to be aware of the cost of poor quality. Be

aware that just because you can't see a problem doesn't mean it's not there. There might even be data that tells you there's a problem, but you either don't have it, can't get it, or don't process it. Sometimes there's the messenger effect, but sometimes there's a powerful interest group within the health system that doesn't want the data to be looked at too closely.

When the data is there but people don't want to see it, I try to bring them on board by pointing out that the information will make everybody's life better. When you improve any process, it protects the patients and the staff without impugning anyone along the way. The data will show your colleagues that you're not making any personal assignments of blame. You're not saying they didn't do a good job ever. When the sample size is good and the statistical testing is good, the numbers speak for themselves, without blaming or attacking anyone.

WORKING IT OUT

In my experience, an organization that commits a lot of type 1 errors really, really wants to be good. This organization has the ability to learn and evolve because it has the motivation. They can be educated to see their errors and move to a calmer approach using statistical process control, not gut feelings. Organizations that commit a lot of type 2 errors are harder to improve. They often don't really want robust data collection and aren't motivated to change.

Organizations aren't usually so clear-cut in their approach to quality improvement. Most commit both type 1 and type 2 errors even while they also get some things right. In the spectrum of problems to have, however, I want an organization that's making mostly type 1 errors. The potential for improvement is much greater.

CHAPTER 10

CHANGES TO MAKE AND CHANGES NOT TO MAKE

It was that time of week again—the hospital administrator and the surgeon were getting together in the little second-floor café for coffee and quality. The hospital administrator had good news: a quality project had just been implemented, and he had high hopes for it.

He told the surgeon, "Remember that issue we were having with changing the ED check-in paperwork so you could see the triage nurse sooner? Once we got past the initial hostility, we put together a good working group. They came up with a lot of improvements, not just for the check-in part, but for the whole triage process. We're working on refining them to make sure they work well. What's that Japanese word you keep using for making things error-proof?"

"Poka-yoke," the surgeon replied. "I prefer to say that rather than idiot-proofing, but error-proofing works, too. Keep an eye out for anything that makes a patient ask a question about the process or not be sure what the answer should be. That's probably a place that needs some poka-yoke attention to make sure the patient gives you the right information without needing help."

The administrator said, "The ED reception clerks and the triage nurses are really excited about this. They gave us a lot of great input based on their experience. The new procedures aren't that different, but I'm hoping those little tweaks take away confusion and let them do the paperwork faster and more accurately. That should make a big difference in moving patients out of the waiting room and triage and into the treatment area faster. If all goes well, we'll be able to celebrate a successful volume to value improvement."

"Nice going," said the surgeon. "Little changes can have a big impact."

✢   ✢   ✢

Catheter-associated urinary-tract infections in hospital-ized patients are considered "never events"—they should never happen. When they do, the hospital is penalized by Medicare and third-party payers. The issue can really burn a hospital. Naturally, hospitals are very interested in ways to avoid UTIs. One hospital I worked at had tried several solutions, and some turned out to be bad choices. They tried taking catheters out of patients before those patients had a chance to develop an infection. That sounds like a good idea because, in general, removing a catheter as early as possible is a good thing, but it's not good if it's removed *too* early. That's an important distinction that didn't get made, and catheters were being removed too early for many patients. In critically ill patients, for instance, the catheter may be needed to follow the patient's urine output carefully. Many ICU patients could not be mon-itored appropriately once their catheters were removed too early. The hospital also tried out perhaps the worst possible solution, which was just not sending samples for urinalysis so they wouldn't have to make the diagnosis. Obviously, that's something we don't want for patients. If a patient gets an infection, we want to know about it and treat it. At this hospital, when patients *did* get a uri-nary-tract infection, it was recognized much later.

BAD AND GOOD SOLUTIONS

In its attempt to solve a problem, the hospital at first chose bad solutions that in some cases actually made patients sicker. Bad solutions often have a certain look about them: they're solutions that are difficult to implement, are expensive, are otherwise prohibitive, take multiple steps to get done, don't work or even backfire, and just generally make things worse.

What do good solutions look like? Above all, a good solution is implementable. A good system makes it easy to do the right thing and hard to make a mistake. A good system is error-proof because the playing field is tilted toward making it easier to do the right thing. In designing the system, the questions are always "What's easy for the physician?" and "What's the right thing for the patient?" and "What's doable?"

THE RIGHT SOLUTION

If a patient comes to the hospital with an existing UTI, then the hospital isn't responsible for it as a hospital-acquired UTI that the patient received in their institution, and therefore the hospital doesn't get penalized. (Of course, the hospital is still responsible for diagnosing and treating the patient properly.) Obviously, the key is to test patients at admission, especially ones who are at high risk, to find out if they already have a catheter-associated UTI. The test is very quick, inexpensive, and easy. To make it a routine part of admissions across the hospital, however, isn't easy. At one hospital where I worked, the center had to decide what changes to make to its system to ensure that every patient, not just the obvious high-risk ones, was automatically tested for a UTI at admission. The solution was fairly obvious: allow nurses to obtain the test, via a standing order from physicians that included certain criteria regarding for who should receive the test and results. The urinanalysis becomes part of a comprehensive outside hospital (jokingly nicknamed the "OSH" for "outside hospital") workup for patients who come from other hospitals, nursing homes, rehab centers, or even retirement communities. These facilities are like "outside hospitals" because their patients are similar to transfers arriving from other hospitals "outside" the one we're describing. This urinalysis test doesn't hurt the patient at all, it's very inexpensive, and there's very little to no downside risk.

This small, simple change turns out to be a big help for the patient and the organization. The comprehensive approach catches not only UTIs but also other problems, such as deep venous thrombosis. That's another condition that can penalize the hospital if the patient develops it during a stay, so it's better to know if they're coming in with it, both to prevent a penalty and to get treatment started right away. Deep venous thrombosis can kill a patient. Part of the OSH workup in the hospital where I worked included a test for deep venous thrombosis.

A good solution is one that is easy to implement, straightforward, and turns out to bolster other quality and safety issues. The best solution makes it easier to do the right thing. In the case of catheter-associated UTIs and deep venous thromboses, the hospital set up standing orders from a physician that empowered ER nurses to order the tests.

USING DATA TO DECIDE

With the DMAIC process—design, measure, analyze, improve, control—you'll often end up with several candidate solutions. How do you filter through the changes that you want to make and the guiding principles to come up with the best solution?

In the case of catheter-related UTIs, you'd want to find a way early in the process to identify patients who arrive with one. You'd want to define what you're measuring. It's very important to align the measurement with the intervention, and vice versa. Are you looking at the percentage of patients who have a urinary-tract infection?

Are you looking at reducing the number of hospitalized patients who have one, measured monthly? The endpoint measurement really matters here, because when you implement the program, you may well see an increased rate of urinary-tract infection in hospitalized patients. That's because now you're looking for them, so you're finding them. But on the other hand, with your new program in place, the rate of hospital-acquired catheter-associated urinary-tract infections should be lower. That leads to a further measurable endpoint: savings from not being penalized by the cost of poor quality.

Part of your UTI rate project may include a SIPOC diagram. Many patients come to the emergency room with catheter-associated infections that they got in their nursing home. So, you can look at nursing homes as suppliers who send you patients. One way to reduce the number of patients coming in with UTIs would be to do outreach to the nursing homes to help them manage catheters better and be more aware of the symptoms of an infection. Or you could do outreach only to the nursing homes that send you the most patients with infections. You could make sure that attending physicians who round on nursing homes are sensitized to the problem. But you also have to be aware of the scope of your project and realize that you can't always influence the people who send you patients. Solutions that work are realistic and within the criteria the team selects.

PAPERWORK PROLIFERATION

Most solutions to quality problems in medicine end up creating more paperwork. I rarely see solutions that involve less paperwork. Based on my experience, I estimate that 80 percent of the solutions that come out of improvement projects typically involve more paperwork—another form to fill out, another item on the chart, another checklist.

I like checklists. They're useful and have a place in quality improvement. But they're only one part of a vast arsenal of what you can do to improve a system. Although checklists are a buzzword and hot topic now, a checklist isn't always the best, most implementable, or most effective solution. It often just creates more paperwork. Checklists can be a good starting point, but they're often not the most effective solution.

Physicians today often spend about half of their working day on paperwork. A checklist that only adds to the load often isn't really helping. For residents, the paperwork is even worse. A lot of it just gets dumped on them, and they end up doing mindless clerical work that doesn't necessarily improve quality. How much of an impact does this have? We don't know, because we don't rigorously measure that sort of work. We don't really know if it makes any difference to quality. We often don't know if we're doing better or worse for having added twenty minutes of paperwork. I advise us all to look to a wider array of interventions than just checklists.

ERROR-PROOFING: THE POKA-YOKE APPROACH

When a system is error-proofed, it's a lot easier for everyone to do the right thing every time and a lot harder to make a mistake. This is the Japanese design philosophy of poka-yoke (pronounced "poke a yoke"), also known as error-proofing, mistake-proofing, or sometimes idiot-proofing. The idea is to set up a system that's as immune to human error as possible. Many mistakes are inadvertent; poka-yoke helps avoid them. In manufacturing processes, where the idea was first developed, poka-yoke is used to prevent mistakes before or while they're being made. The idea is to eliminate defects at the source.

For example, on an assembly line, a poka-yoke solution to putting a part in backward might be to redesign it so that it can only fit when it's in the proper position, or to color it on one side so that you can see immediately if it's in place correctly. If a part requires the worker to install five screws, provide the screws in packages of five so that forgetting one or using the wrong screw becomes almost impossible.

In healthcare, where we're dealing with humans in fluid situations that require experience and judgment, poka-yoke changes aren't generally as easy as just retooling a part. For example, although we commonly use kits that contain everything needed for a procedure such as inserting a central line, often the procedure doesn't require everything in the kit, leaving plenty of room for human error. In medicine, we have to make it easier to do the right thing even when the right thing is complex and the people who need to do it are very busy and have a lot of distractions. Under these circumstances, poka-yoke solutions almost always mean making something harder, either mechanically, physically, mentally, structurally, or by creating more paperwork. This sounds counterproductive and more like punishment than help, but in fact, by making it harder to deviate from a process or protocol, the system makes it harder to mess up. Great healthcare poka-yoke solutions are ones that eliminate or reduce the ability to make a mistake *and* eliminate some piece of paperwork!

Some poka-yoke solutions are very simple, such as pop-up messages on a computer screen or making a form easier to fill in correctly by highlighting where the information needs to go. A good example of a simple poka-yoke solution for hand cleanliness is simply putting hand-sanitizer dispensers outside every doorway. If you have to look around for a dispenser, you might skip sanitizing; if a dispenser is right in front of you everywhere you turn, you'll probably use it.

Processes and protocols are there for a reason: we know they lead to the best outcomes. Poka-yoke changes tilt the playing field and make it easier to stick to doing the right thing. Ideally, a poka-yoke change in a medical system makes something happen the right way automatically, without anyone really noticing that they've been guided in the right direction.

Let's say you're focused on identifying patients in the ED who are critically ill and need to get to the intensive-care unit quickly. You collect the data and find that some patient populations aren't being flagged as critically ill soon enough. These populations are underrecognized as being at particular risk: elderly patients who are septic, immunosuppressed patients, morbidly obese patients, other patients who don't always appear to be as sick as they really are—you're missing them. You want to make changes that will make it easier for the ED staff to recognize these patients sooner.

At the same time, the staff in the intensive-care unit are very busy all the time; the unit doesn't have enough beds. To protect themselves and make sure only the patients who really need to be in intensive care get sent there, the staff has erected a lot of barriers. They've set up a lot of different criteria that the ED staff has to meet to get a patient admitted to their ICU.

The problem is, the ED criteria for intensive care and the ICU criteria for admission aren't aligned. The ED criteria don't make it easy to discover the patients who need critical care. They're underrecognized. At the same time, the criteria for the critical-care unit make it hard to admit a patient there. The issue is how to adapt the criteria at both ends to tilt the field. How can you error-proof both parts of the hospital to make sure patients who need critical care don't get missed in the ED and are admitted quickly to the ICU?

One poka-yoke way is to create an exception for certain groups of patients. You change the admission criteria to the critical-care unit for these subpopulations. When you carve those groups out, you have less chance of overlooking them. They're automatically candidates for intensive care without having to fill out additional paperwork or get someone to authorize it.

You have to put procedures in place that make the right thing more likely to happen. It won't always happen, because we're dealing with human beings, both staff and patients. Sometimes we're not sure what the diagnosis is and can't tell how sick the patient is. Sometimes doctors misdiagnose or disagree with each other on the diagnosis. Ideally, for ICU admission, a physician would stay by the bedside of a patient until there's a conversation between the physician and the ICU attending physician about whether this patient should go to the unit or not. That's not hard-core error proofing, because it's still possible to have a defect from human error, but it makes it less likely. Realistically, however, because of time demands, diagnostic uncertainty, waiting for test results, uncooperative patients, and much more, we can't always achieve total error-proofing. But as you know from the rest of this book, that's *not* to say there isn't huge potential to deliver higher quality care in medicine.

As another example, you want to make sure that all medication is administered correctly. The system is set up to avoid mistakes. Each time a medication is given to a patient, it first has to be vetted by the electronic medical record and the patient's nurse; this is done by scanning the patient's electronic bracelet and the medicine container in addition to a review process. If the bracelet and container don't match, an alert appears. The computer checks for whether the patient has an allergy to the medication or any similar medication. Other steps proceed. The nurse or aide has to ask the patient his or her name and date of birth before giving the medication to make sure it's going to the right person. These steps are all built in to the routine of giving medications in such a way that they're almost impossible to skip.

Upstream, when the doctor prescribes the medication using the computerized entry system, the computer flags any possible allergies or dangerous interactions. It's possible to override or ignore the red flags, but many safeguards make sure the right patient is getting the right medications and prevent entering the wrong medication or wrong dose. Of course, you can't eliminate every possible drug error completely, but you can get pretty close.

With good error-proofing, defects are hard to create because the process can't move on to the next step unless previous steps are perfect. Some will still slip through, simply because so many patients are getting so many medications with so many possible interactions with other medications. To me, the amazing thing is that more errors don't happen, but to the health-care consumer (and me as their doctor), any error is a big problem. The reality is that a lot of things have to go wrong in a row for a serious medication error to occur. Given the sheer volume of events, mistakes will inevitably happen.

Again, let me say that a recognition that events will happen does *not* mean we are unable to lower the event rate we currently see. A typical event rate in a service industry is one defect per one thousand opportunities at making a defect. The pursuit with tools such as those seen in Lean Six Sigma is the reduction of defects to 3.4 defects per one million opportunities at making a defect. I include that as a reminder that we have a *lot* of room to improve, even while we recognize that things happen.

IMPLEMENTING ERROR-PROOFING

Poka-yoke design ideas are really about "implementability." We change processes to make them mistake-proof. That makes them easier to do, gives better outcomes, and avoids errors. Making those changes in a way that helps, not hinders, takes knowing what the people on the front line think the right thing is. You need to talk to the people using the system—the end users, the people at the tip of the spear.

When you unpack poka-yoke, it includes elements of end-user design. What do the people at the tip of the spear think? They're the ones who are implementing the strategies and participating in the system, so you've got to listen to them. Because they use the systems every day, they already have a pretty good idea of where things are likely to go wrong, why, and what to do about it. They have to be the ones to tell you what will work. A top-down management approach that imposes a change is one of the least effective approaches. In fact, that approach is almost completely incompatible with poka-yoke, which relies on suggestions from the people actually doing the work. Show them the system data and performance, and ask them what they think can be done to make it easier to do better.

Some of the best-functioning organizations in the business world have the least number of formal policies. They've designed many safeguard procedures into the usual processes so that they don't have to be written down or imposed from the top. They're already in place and part of the company culture.

I don't think you can run a health-care system without formal policies—quite the opposite, in fact. But when you want to implement poka-yoke changes, the people affected have to be in the room as stakeholders to tell you if the change would make it easier for them to do the right thing. Not all poka-yoke changes need to be written as policies. You have to listen, which isn't always easy. Poka-yoke changes can be a tough conversation. Staff members may not want to accept a change that forces them to follow a procedure in a certain way or makes it harder to deviate from a protocol. That can make them feel as if their clinical judgment is being questioned or their autonomy is being limited. But having those tough, difficult conversations is crucial. The mark of a good organization is to be able to have those conversations collegially. When you really listen, you'll hear the staff say, "I want quality, too. I didn't show up to work today to do a bad job, but I don't have the resources I need to get some things done right." Some health-care organizations have cut so deeply that the staff lack basic resources. These kinds of meetings, where people vent their frustrations with the system, can be very difficult. One solution would be finding more resources, but the reality is often that the resources aren't there and they're not coming any time soon. That doesn't mean you can't be creative and make improvements. Not everything needs resources and money thrown at it.

You often can make meaningful changes just with simple modifications of existing procedures. Although the resource issue tends to lurk behind multiple quality problems and constricts potential solutions, that doesn't mean you can't do anything. If you implement three or four inexpensive changes that each decrease the probability of a defect, you soon have little money spent and *many* fewer defects made.

One of the criteria you evaluate solutions against is "implementability." If the solution can't be implemented, it can be the best solution of all time, but it doesn't matter. One of the barriers to implementation is simple lack of funds. If no capital for some change is available, then just cross that particular solution off the list. Go to the ones that need imagination, not money, to work. Problems only rarely have just one solution.

A small input can have a big impact down the line. To return to the UTI example, if you immediately treat a patient with a UTI on admission, that's likely to make the patient feel better and lead to a shorter hospital stay. It's easy to do and very inexpensive, and it can lead to huge cost savings by avoiding complications. That's what a good solution looks like. We can easily quantify it by tracking changes in detection and discharge times and correlating them. We can even help our patients after discharge by identifying the nursing homes that are most likely to send a patient with a UTI and simply notifying them that their UTI rate is high compared to other nursing homes in the area. That's not difficult or expensive, yet it can have a big impact down the line.

Another good example is placing peripherally inserted central catheter (PICC) lines. The infection rate for these is now very low. We've developed poka-yoke protocols that make sterile procedure much easier to follow when inserting the lines. We've also developed better protocols for deciding who really needs to have these devices and getting them out as soon as they're not needed anymore.

CHANGES NOT TO MAKE

Changes not to make include those that are very expensive or are outside the control of the group. Any change that will take too long to implement, or is beyond the scope of the quality-improvement project and data collection, shouldn't be made. If you focus the discussion in advance on what a good solution looks like, you're a lot less likely to propose a change that shouldn't be made. If the change doesn't fit with the good solution, don't do it.

CHAPTER 11

HOW TO KNOW IF YOU'RE REALLY DOING BETTER

Months of regular weekly coffee meetings had gone by; the hospital administrator and the surgeon had both helped initiate a number of quality-improvement projects. For the earliest projects, it was getting to be time to review the results and decide if the project was a success. The hospital administrator was getting nervous.

"How am I supposed to know when to declare success?" he asked the surgeon. "I'm worried that some of the project results

look better than they really are. In fact, I'm pretty sure one of them isn't working out at all, even though the dashboard numbers are looking better."

The surgeon answered, "This is when Lean Six Sigma statistical testing really comes in. If you did everything right up until now, especially with your data sampling, you should be able to tell from the statistical process-control tools if you've really accomplished anything. Chances are you did, but it might not be what you think. Only the numbers can tell you for sure."

+ + +

You've seen it before in this book: statistical testing is the key to knowing if you're really doing better as a result of your quality-improvement project. In healthcare, it's easy to think you're doing better even when you're not. You can't throw the party until you're sure you're doing better from a statistically valid standpoint. (Well, you *can*, of course. I just recommend you don't.) Statistical testing tells you whether the team is doing better and the system as a whole is doing better. You can't rely on subjective data based on how well a few cases went after you made a change. You're happy, but until you see some numbers, you can't say the system is doing any better than it did before.

Remember, this is especially true of low-probability events such as wound infections. These are pretty unusual events in hospitals, so focusing on reducing their frequency doesn't really change anything. The hospital could go three months without any wound infections, but the rate is so low to begin with that this number is almost meaningless. It's just as likely that they got lucky as it is that a system change made any difference.

We tend to confuse motion with activity and success. In the case of wound infections, the protocols might get changed, which is motion, and then for the next three months the infection rate, already very low, might drop to zero. Everybody feels great about it, but the motion hasn't led to true success. Just because something is moving doesn't mean it's achieving anything. In golf, you can have a lot of activity—you could take ten swings to get the ball in the hole and think you've achieved success. You have, in the sense that you eventually got the ball in the hole, but the idea is to do it with the least number of swings.

If you get to know a little bit about process improvement and statistical process control, you can't really fool yourself anymore. You'll avoid making changes that don't accomplish anything. Your heart might be in the right place, but without statistics, even if you're working really hard, you won't be getting anywhere. That's very common in healthcare. It's a problem for people, because it's depressing to work so hard and see no results, or even worse, to realize you were tampering with the system and made things worse. Use the approaches in this book to focus on value and quality delivery in a way that makes sure you aren't spinning your wheels.

HAND WASHING

In healthcare, we're kind of fanatical about hand washing. We want everyone washing their hands or using hand sanitizer all the time as the best way to prevent spreading illness and infections. The higher the rate of hand washing, the happier we are and the healthier our patients are. Most importantly, when staff wash their hands a lot, we believe the rate of Methicillin-resistant Staphylococcus aureus (MRSA) infections goes down. Since these infections are extremely serious and sometimes fatal, anything that increases the hand-washing rate is good, right?

At one hospital, we started a program to encourage hand washing among the staff. We were successful: hand washing rates shot up to 80 percent in one month. Was this a victory? Yes, but it wasn't as impressive as it sounds: the starting rate was 75 percent. In fact, you could look at the program as something of a failure, because it only got the rate up to 80 percent. And if you don't know the starting rate and how big the sample was, you can't really say if there was any improvement. And, guess what? That 5 percent change wasn't significant. We were just as good (or bad?) at hand washing as we ever were.

The question I always ask myself isn't, "Am I doing better?" I like to ask myself instead, "When can I celebrate? When can I say, 'Awesome job, everybody?'" What I don't want to say is, "We're doing a little less badly because of our quality-improvement project." I want to say, "Wow, this is really great."

We actually can get a pretty good idea of things like hand washing rates among hospital personnel by using silent observers from the quality-improvement staff. They're well known to the staff—what they do isn't a secret or hidden. As part of quality-improvement projects, they walk around on the hospital floors. They might take a sample of ten patient encounters several times a day. They get a good sense of things like how many times a physician completely washed their hands before seeing the patient. They used a standard definition: they washed all surfaces for at least ten seconds with soap and water, not alcohol gel.

This sort of observation is sometimes done on a routine basis just to make sure everyone is on the ball about hand washing. Sometimes it's done because we suspect there's a problem. I like to align observation with the importance of the outcome. Every patient-care issue is important, but every hospital has certain things they're better at or worse at. Some hospitals need their financial department to be better. Some need their quality to be better. Often those two are intertwined. Deploying silent observers isn't a good use of resources if the problem isn't really observable on the floor.

A hospital always needs something improved. If you pick a quality-improvement project, whether it's hand washing or something else, you have to start with a sense of how good the current process is. You don't have any data yet, so you need to think about how important your project is to the organizational mission. Do you need to do a full project to improve something? These projects take a while, and the time they take from people maybe could be better used elsewhere. In the case of the improved hand-washing statistic, we needed real data directly from the process. We needed to have people stand there silently with a clipboard, timing how often and for how long people washed their hands. The data is collected anonymously—we don't take staff or patient names. We wanted to know what our people were doing on the spot, rather than relying on data from other hospitals and other studies.

Once you have a snapshot of how your system is working, that's powerful. It shows you that maybe you're not doing as well as you thought. Rarely, it shows that you're doing much better than you think. That's why data are key. It teaches you not to take anything for granted. Even if you think things are going well, you still need to look at the data.

Let's go back to the example of zero tolerance for wound infections. You're already doing better than you were and better than the hospital down the street and better than the national average. But you don't want to be just average. You want to be excellent. That's one good reason to look at your data often—to get from good to great. But at the same time, if the data consistently shows you're doing really well, maybe you can shift your focus to other areas.

GETTING THE RIGHT SAMPLE SIZE

If you want to see if you're really doing well with something or if you're just fooling yourself, you need to have a large enough sample size to be able to tell the difference. Often, however, getting a large enough sample size could take too long. If you think your data endpoint is going to take a year to get, for example, and making a change is going to take another year after that, that's probably way too slow. You can work around this by selecting a data endpoint that is both meaningful and that you can get in a reasonable amount of time. Look for something that's a surrogate for the larger endpoint, something that you think is associated with it closely enough that you can get a good sense of where you are before you get to the endpoint. Pick a reasonable data point that you think has meaning and can show reasonable change in a reasonable amount of time. Pick your shot carefully.

For example, in the case of surgical wound infections in clean surgical wounds (which are rare), your data are discrete. The patient either gets a wound infection or doesn't. With such a low number of infections, it's going to take you forever to get enough patients in the sample to see a meaningful change. And the number is already pretty good, which makes it even more difficult.

Rather than try to get enough discrete data to discover anything of importance, try a different, nonbinary approach. You can't collect enough yes/no infection data, but you can score the process of preventing wound infections. Were the procedures for preventing infection followed? Was the skin prepped properly? Was the operative time appropriate, or did the case take longer than routine because of some factor? Did the patient get the right pre-op antibiotics, and was the patient redosed if necessary? Did we properly identify the case?

You could come up with a scoring system for how well you're doing these procedures, and then you could score twenty random cases. Now you've converted a discrete data endpoint into a more continuous data endpoint that can show motion and might identify areas that could be improved with better procedures or a change to the checklist.

CHAPTER 12

YOUR TEAM FUMBLED AT THE ONE-YARD LINE: CHANGES THAT DON'T STICK

A few more months went by. Overall, the hospital administrator and the surgeon were both pleased with most of their quality-improvement projects. They had demonstrably helped move the hospital in the direction of value over volume. But lately, over their weekly coffee meeting in the little second-floor café, the hospital administrator admitted that doubts were starting to creep in. Most of his projects seemed to improve things, but he had noticed that some of the improvements weren't sticking.

"Our ED admissions project shaved ten minutes off the time it took to get through the check-in and triage processes, but last time I checked, the time was creeping back up again. I can't figure out why," he told the surgeon. "Those control charts are really confusing."

"They are a little hard to understand," the surgeon agreed. "Get your Lean Six Sigma black belt to take a look at them. It could be you need a different type of chart, or maybe you just need to adjust the variance on your control points so you see a problem happening sooner. You also need to look beyond the chart, because all that tells you is what's happening, not why it's happening. Lots of external factors, such as personnel changes, can keep a change from sticking. If you set up the control chart so you can get on them right away if they start to drift backward, you have a better chance of making the changes last."

✛　✛　✛

Back in chapter 8 I talked about a healthcare organization that wasn't doing well with supervised resident positions. They didn't document the supervision well, so they couldn't tell if the residents were really being supervised adequately or not. They decided to study the process. They did a good study, with an appropriate sample size. However, they started out on the wrong foot by collecting discrete data. They asked only, "Was the resident supervised, yes or no?" They realized their mistake quickly and changed the data collection to make it continuous. They followed the strategies I've outlined in this book. They collected data, they made changes, and they made significant improvement in resident supervision.

The months passed, and gradually, without anyone really noticing, resident supervision backslid. The team had fumbled at the one-yard line. They'd done great work, but they couldn't sustain it. Part of the reason was that once the new system was put in place, everyone just assumed it would work well and keep running by itself. The quality team didn't check in on it. Over time, systems tend to change, atrophy, and break down—the resident supervision system was no different. When the hospital switched to electronic records, the resident supervision part of the patient chart wasn't reviewed. It turned out to be hard to use in the electronic format, but nobody really noticed that the records were getting sloppy. They found out only because six months afterward, someone thought to say, "Hey, remember we did this project? I wonder how that's going?" When they looked at it, they went, "Oh, my gosh," and tuned it up to work better with the new records system.

That wasn't being systematic, however—it was just luck.

THE LAST YARD

The final part of a quality-improvement project is setting it up so you get feedback from the system on a regular basis. If you don't do that last part correctly, you don't know that things have gone haywire until a problem jumps out at you. All quality-improvement projects need a control phase that lets the system signal you and tell you when things aren't going right anymore. All the work you did on your quality-improvement project isn't really over until you answer the final question, "How do we sustain improvement?"

The answer is by using the right tools in the control phase. In healthcare, patients come through the system one at a time, but to get the big picture, Lean Six Sigma often uses control charts after the quality-improvements have been implemented. All a control chart can tell you is that a system is functioning at its routine level of performance over time. It can't tell you whether that routine level of performance is acceptable or not. If you look only at the control chart (especially if you do that too early), everything may look as if it's going fine, but in fact, the performance may be totally unacceptable. This is why control charts shouldn't be applied until the end of a quality project: although the control chart can tell us when the system is performing routinely, it can lull us to sleep, because that routine may be no good.

Control charts vary, depending on what you're measuring and how your data is distributed. Your Lean Six Sigma black belt is the right person to help you decide which type of chart to use and understand what it's telling you. You would use a different control for averages over time than you would for proportions over time, for example. In healthcare, we often use a control chart that tracks individuals as they come through the system. It's called an individual moving range (IMR) chart. It plots patients and people or events as they come through the system one at a time. The range is an important part of the IMR chart. Range is a measure of variance between data points. In other words, range shows you how wide the swings are in your data. If you see an unusual amount of variance between data points, the question becomes "Why is there such a wide swing? What is it telling us?"

APPLYING THE RULES

If you don't build a control chart into the ongoing phase of your quality-improvement project, and look at it on a regular basis, you won't pick up the signals that say, "This case is beyond the upper control level. Something must have gotten out of whack with this case. We have to look into it." The power of the control chart is that it will tell you when things are going off the rails.

To understand what's going on with your control charts, Lean Six Sigma applies what are known as the Shewart Rules, which are rooted in the Westinghouse Rules originally devised by Westinghouse Electric. The rules tell what to look for in the control charts to see if a problem is on the way or is already there. Often, obvious signs tell you about a problem. A data point might be above or below the limits set in the chart. In healthcare, we mostly look for variants above the limit, because that often indicates that something took too long or didn't go smoothly. If something is more than three standards deviations beyond what's expected, that means there's less than a 1 percent chance that it happened at random. You need to look into it.

Control charts need to be checked on a regular schedule, but they also need to be reviewed if anything external changes the system. The chief of the department might leave as part of personnel shuffle. That means new people come in who may not understand the system well. The control chart should be checked more often to see where the personnel changes may be affecting quality. A lot can change quickly in just a month or two. The control phase provides feedback from the system when something has gone wrong, or something needs maintenance, or the weeds need trimming.

SUSTAINING THE GAINS

At one hospital, the goal of the quality-improvement project was to reduce turnaround time in the operating rooms. The staff worked hard and got the turnaround times much lower. But only three months later, the turnaround time had crept back up again to where it had been. Because where it had been was actually pretty good, nobody noticed at first that the turnaround times were slowing down from great to just good again, until one day the OR got very backed up because a couple of turnarounds took forty minutes. The chief surgeon wasn't happy and didn't hesitate to tell anyone he could how he felt.

What had kept the gains from being sustained? A combination of factors. Two new people started in the OR; one longtime employee in the facilities-service department had retired. The new people weren't educated about the turnaround system, but that wasn't the real problem. The quality-improvement team hadn't built a control plan into the system. The only way they knew they had a problem was when the chief surgeon fired off an angry e-mail to the administration and most of the staff.

IS IT THE PLAN?

Sometimes an improvement doesn't stick because it's not a good improvement. You can't just tweak it; it's back to the drawing board. When a situation starts to slide backward, you might not be able to tell right away, even if you have the right control chart. Normal variation in the data can hide an insidious problem for a long time. This is where data can be so powerful. It's hard to see the big picture when you're focused on just your aspect of it. Often people tell you what they think you want to hear, and you're so busy that you don't question it. The data keeps you from being misled by letting you review the whole system without bias. It shows you when the system is experiencing normal variation and when it's actually worsening. The data may let you see when the system isn't running according to a normal bell curve with reliably good numbers but instead is shifting in one direction.

One key goal of Lean Six Sigma is to decrease the variation in a system. You want to be able to fit six standard deviations of data between the lowest limit the customer would accept (the lower specification limit) and the upper limit that's acceptable to the customer (the upper specification limit).

The upper control limit in a system, as seen on a control chart, is typically defined as three standard deviations away from the mean. Choosing the right control chart and analyzing the data from it can be complicated, especially if the data isn't normally distributed—as it can often be in healthcare. Your Lean Six Sigma black belt is the person to work with to set up the chart and teach you how to interpret the data.

Bear in mind that the lower and upper specification limit is *not* the same as a lower or upper control limit on a control chart. The upper specification limit (USL) comes from what the customer will accept. The upper control limit (UCL) comes from what the data demonstrate as (typically) three standard deviations away from the central tendency of the data. That's why a control chart can *only* tell us whether the system is performing as expected. A control chart *can't* tell us whether that system is performing in a way that is acceptable. (For examples of control charts, check my blog at surgicalbusinessmodelinnovation. com/?s=control+chart.)

IMPLEMENTING THE CONTROL PHASE

Making sure the control phase gets implemented and maintained is crucial to the long-term sustainability of your quality improvements. When I'm the black belt, I like to specifically designate an individual on the project team to be the person who's given the data, makes the control chart, and lets everyone know how it's going. Responsibility for the project then gets baked into that person's job description, so if he leaves, his replacement automatically takes over, including getting any necessary training.

Before I leave the project, I educate the team about what could go wrong. I teach them what red flags to look for, what problems they can fix on their own, and what problems they should call me about right away. Giving the process back to the people who own it is called *repatriating*. I like to make someone in the group that lives with the process every day responsible for monitoring it and alerting the person she reports to if the data go awry. The problem has to be immediately passed up the chain. If I get a report that the wheels are coming off the bus, I want input from the group about how to fix it. It took a group to make the improvement, and it's going to take a group to repair it.

I usually start by asking the group, "What do you think is wrong? Did anything change? What happened?" If the answer isn't very clear and a change isn't easy to implement, then we need the group to meet more to figure it out.

The control phase is the capstone to a quality-improvement project. It's the key to sustaining improvement. It's essential, not just nice to have, but it's not the most fulfilling part of a project. Not every organization gets there with every project. An organization that's new to quality improvement through Lean Six Sigma might make it past the goal line in only about a third of their first projects. With experience, however, I find that about 90 percent of projects are successful. With experience and patience, quality-improvement projects go well and have lasting results.

CONCLUSION

USE THE TOOLS

That's the road map to go from volume of services provided to value for patients. It's quantitative, and it takes sophistication with data, along with aligned culture. The process is *not* easy, but it is *very* fulfilling for providers, administrators, and—most importantly—patients.

In this book, I've talked about successes and failures with quality-improvement projects. I've explained how using Lean Six Sigma techniques gives you real, actionable data that can help tilt the odds in favor of success. I've been privileged to use these tools with a number of institutions that have made tremendous improvements in quality, as measured by items that are important to patients and third-party payers. It has been amazing and fulfilling to see how transformative these tools can be when deployed meaningfully.

When the tools are used correctly, the impact is large. In one system, we even saw an increase in patient volume without any increase in friction within the system—in fact, quality improved. The system was able to help more people in a robust, high-quality way. It turned out that a higher quality process provided more value and allowed us to help more patients. That system was one of volume *and* value.

IMPROVING ACUTE-CARE SURGERY

I was also able to use Lean Six Sigma tools to revitalize the trauma and acute-care surgery section of a large hospital. We were able to increase patient volume while delivering care that was very high quality. We didn't just think we were providing excellent quality—we demonstrated it with improved data. As measured by compliance with national and state standards, the revitalization process created high-quality outcomes that surpassed standards.

The section had a low-volume trauma program. When patients did come through it, the results weren't very good—the cases often didn't seem to go right. Part of the problem was a separate issue of initial care in the ED, before the patient was sent for surgery. The ED staff wasn't supervised well, and documentation was poor. More importantly, the patient care wasn't timely. Physicians weren't seeing patients soon enough, to the point where the ED was often out of compliance with guidelines. Sick patients weren't being identified as sick in a timely way; they weren't being admitted to the hospital soon enough.

The hospital had tried a lot of quick fixes, but they didn't have any data to show the fixes were helping. I was brought in to help improve the overall situation. The process took several months, as these projects often do. We followed the DMAIC approach. We were able to refocus and improve, in a statistically significant fashion, almost everything done for patients, starting at the front door of the hospital. The team focused on data rather than culture issues. Because the staff were at odds with each other over some cultural points, focusing on the data took those issues out of the picture.

The data-driven approach focused on using continuous data with the DMAIC project. We started with a very good project charter that emphasized the cost support benefit of quality improvement. We used clear operational definitions. We made a SIPOC diagram and used it to create a solid data-collection plan. We made changes only when we had enough data with a big enough sample size to show current performance. The changes were mostly focused on poka-yoke principles of making it easier to do the right thing every time.

After each change was made, we collected data again to see if it actually worked and where it could be improved. The changes made it easier to see patients quickly and easier to document the good work that was already being done in the ED. Each of those tools conspired to make improvements happen fast, without a lot of disruption. Such was the power of data that the emergency department became very compliant very quickly. The outcomes from trauma surgery improved. The ED started to grow, without the sort of friction that rapid growth can bring to a system. It's a great success story because the team used the Lean Six Sigma tools.

One reason this project succeeded so well is that we avoided scope creep, a common reason quality-improvement projects fail. We were very aware of this possibility and deliberately kept the scope of the project very narrowly focused on the front door of the ED. The project started the clock as the call came in that the ambulance was on its way; the clock stopped when the patient physically got to his or her post-ED destination.

We were very clear about the operational definitions. The original thinking was that the clock would stop when the order went into the computer to discharge the patient or transfer him or her from the ED to a hospital bed. That wasn't a good idea, because patients were often still in the ED for hours after their orders went in. This is where the power of the Lean Six Sigma tools showed very clearly: it brought all the stakeholders together to come up with much better, very clear operational definitions of what *discharge* and *transfer* really meant. When everyone agreed on the definitions, then the data points and how to collect them also became very clear. Finally, what constituted victory also became very clear.

In this project, the control phase was really key. Because the changes were made in a very measurable and robust way that had clear positive impact, they stuck—and kept going in the right direction for years after they were first implemented. If an issue arose in the system, the programmed-in control phase would signal the providers and the Lean Six Sigma black belt. We could then look in on it, see where the problem was, and fix it, almost always very quickly.

CORRECTING OVERCORRECTING

I worked with the surgery department of a large hospital

to get them out of a cycle of consistent type 1 errors. They were overcorrecting and overcontrolling for problems that really weren't problems. They were focusing on the wrong things, which led to the staff working harder but not smarter.

By having the quality-improvement team focus on data, they were able to move away from culture and political issues. In Lean Six Sigma statistical process control, the data doesn't have a name—nobody is attached to it. Lean Six Sigma helps prevent type 1 and type 2 errors by sticking to the data instead of gut feelings. When working with this team, we had some very valuable discussions about type 1 and type 2 errors. Just as valuable was the stakeholder and team-based approach to data collection, analysis, and selection of improvements. It was very fulfilling to see how Lean Six Sigma techniques were able to realign the whole department and allow for growth. The new systems are robust and have good process control built into them. It's a bit soon to tell how long-lasting the changes will be, but I'm very optimistic. In my experience, when a department starts to move down the quality-improvement path in a very organized, focused, and data-driven way, the improvements stick. That old saying, "Well begun is half done," really applies to quality improvement.

PATIENT BENEFITS

Even a quality-improvement project that seems remote from patient care, such as an initiative to cut waste in the operating room, benefits patients in the long run. At the end of the scalpel, at the top of the pyramid, there's always a patient. When we do a quality-improvement project that helps reduce ventilator-associated pneumonia, for instance, that may mean a shorter hospital stay and probably a better outcome for a individual patient. But it also means more bed availability in the intensive-care unit for other patients; that means the physicians, nurses, and staff members can help more patients. The cost savings to Medicare and third-party payers are substantial when a patient gets off the ventilator quickly and without any complications.

CALL ME

Quality-improvement projects using Lean Six Sigma have a cost, but the potential payoff almost always offsets the expense many times over. It's a tool set that can be used to build a garden shed or a house, a rowboat or a yacht—whatever the organization needs. Still, it's often hard for a healthcare organization to understand how these tools protect patients, improve the quality of decisions, and improve hospital systems. Our training as physicians tends to make us focus on dramatic events and outliers rather than on overall quality. We'll adjust an entire system because of a single event, since that event really gets our attention, while ignoring or being unable to see the real messages the system is sending. In some ways, our tendency to want to correct what is in front of us unfortunately worsens the quality in the system as a whole.

Quality-improvement projects in healthcare have the best chance of success if they're carefully planned using the Lean Six Sigma tools. This takes some special expertise, which is why the Lean Six Sigma approach, effective as it is, isn't used as much as it could and should be in healthcare. Some approaches are very straightforward and easy to apply; others aren't. Some big systems grow their own Lean Six Sigma experts, but for most, the best way to get lasting quality improvement is to bring in a Lean Six Sigma black belt right at the start to help with a one-off project or to set up a system for training their own crop of local experts.

When an experienced facilitator is brought in to manage the project and help crunch the numbers, it removes a big pain point for the members of the team. Now they don't have to do one of the most difficult aspects of the project, and they can be sure the calculations will be done correctly and produce reliable results. If there's someone doing all that work behind the scenes for you, you're more willing to participate in the project and put your own talents to their best use.

THESURGICALLAB.COM

I'm always interested in helping health-care systems improve their quality with Lean Six Sigma tools. Whether you just want to know a bit more, want training for your in-house specialists, are ready to bring in a black belt for a large project, or are interested in a training session on quality, I'm here to help. Get in touch with me at dmkashmer@thesurgicallab.com. I'm always happy to answer questions and share ideas.

RESOURCES

THEHEALTHCAREQUALITYPODCAST.COM

Here's the home for our audio and video podcasts focused on the use of statistical process-control tools in healthcare. You can also find the podcasts on iTunes and Sound-Cloud. A link to the podcasts and other related links is at TheSurgicalLab.com.

THEHEALTHCAREQUALITYBLOG.COM

I've maintained this blog for several years. This site provides entries on quality improvement in healthcare using statistical process-control tools, podcast transcripts, and links to useful content. The focus is on quality-improvement tools and their applications in healthcare. Related topics include business-model innovation in healthcare.

THE HIDDEN CURRICULUM: WHAT THEY DON'T TEACH YOU AT MEDICAL SCHOOL

This book focuses on useful information for physicians (especially surgeons) that doctors aren't taught in medical school. In particular, chapter 8 focuses on important points about how data is used to evaluate health-care providers. The book is available at TheHiddenCurriculum.company.

BLOG.MINITAB.COM

Minitab has a software product that's very helpful for Lean Six Sigma statistical analysis. The blog is *great*. It focuses on very practical information about how to apply advanced quality tools to fields such as healthcare. Each entry highlights different tools and how to apply them with the Minitab software product. Although there are many different software tools available for quality improvement in healthcare, Minitab is one of my favorites.

INSIGHTS.THESURGICALLAB.COM

I use this site to share brief updates on hot topics related to health-care quality improvement in a social-media friendly format.

AMERICAN SOCIETY FOR QUALITY

The American Society for Quality offers a lot of good information on its website, ASQ.org.

PRACTICAL LEAN SIX SIGMA FOR HEALTHCARE: USING THE A3 AND LEAN THINKING TO IMPROVE OPERATIONAL PERFORMANCE IN HOSPITALS, CLINICS, AND PHYSICIAN GROUP PRACTICES

This book by Todd Sperl et al. (MCS Media, Inc., 2013) is an excellent guide to Lean Six Sigma in healthcare. It is available at Amazon.com.

ABOUT THE AUTHOR

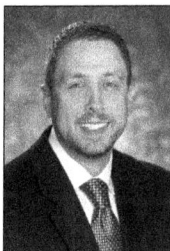

DR. DAVID KASHMER is the Chief of Surgical Services at Signature Healthcare, as well as a trauma and acute-care surgeon. He earned his Medical Doctor degree from MCP Hahnemann University—now Drexel University College of Medicine—and his Bachelor of Science degree in biology from Villanova University through a joint BS-MD program with MCP Hahnemann.

He also earned a Lean Six Sigma master black belt certificate at Villanova. Kashmer holds a Master of Business Administration degree in Healthcare Administration from George Washington University.